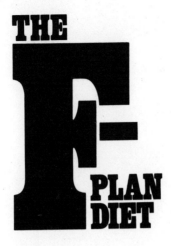

THE F-PLAN DIET

THE F-PLAN DIET

AUDREY EYTON

BANTAM BOOKS

TORONTO · NEW YORK · LONDON · SYDNEY

THE F-PLAN DIET

A Bantam Book/March 1983

All rights reserved.
Copyright © 1982, 1983 by Audrey Eyton
This book may not be reproduced, in whole or in part, by mimeograph or any other means, without permission. For information address: Bantam Books, Inc.

    Library of Congress Cataloging in Publication Data
    Eyton, Audrey.
      The F-Plan diet.
      Includes index.
      1. Reducing diets.   2. High-fiber diet.
    I. Title.
    RM222.2.E97   1983   613.2   82-17969
    ISBN: 0-553-05038-9

Published simultaneously in Canada by Bantam Books, Inc. and in the United States by Crown Publishers, Inc.

Bantam Books are published by Bantam Books, Inc. Its trademark, consisting of the words "Bantam Books" and the portrayal of a rooster, is Registered in U.S. Patent and Trademark Office and in other countries. Marca Registrada. Bantam Books, Inc., 666 Fifth Avenue, New York, New York 10103.

Printed in the United States of America

9   8   7

Contents

Acknowledgments

I would like to express my gratitude to Derek Miller and Dr. Elizabeth Evans of London University for their invaluable help and guidance in the research and testing of the F-Plan diet, and, in the United States, to my longtime friend Dr. Theodore van Itallie of St. Luke's Hospital in New York City, and to Dr. James W. Anderson, director of the Veterans Medical Service, Lexington, Kentucky, and his assistant, Mrs. Beverly Seiling, for providing charts giving dietary fiber content in foods popular with Americans, in familiar measurements for realistic serving portions.

My warmest thanks to Betty Wason, American home economist and cookbook author, who "Americanized" recipes from the British edition of *The F-Plan Diet*, using American ingredient measures, and added recipes of her own.

I

THE F-PLAN

Introduction

Over the past years, many claims have been made suggesting that the inclusion of some particular food in a diet would specifically help overweight people lose weight more quickly and effectively. Grapefruit is one example. Grapefruit diets were popular for years. Then pineapple was said to be invested with magical weight-shedding powers. Steak or other meats consumed several times a day have also been promoted as a wonderfully quick way to slim down. Sadly, all such claims about the value of one particular food or food element were based on fiction rather than fact—certainly not on any established medical fact. No substance we eat has been proved by scientific methods to have any realistic effect in speeding away our surplus fat. Weight loss depended entirely on calories we *didn't* eat.

But now, for the first time in the history of medical science, a natural food substance has been isolated about which it can be said: *If you base your reducing diet on this food element you should lose weight more quickly and easily than with the same calorie total of other foods.* And this diet has the backing of medical science.

The substance is dietary fiber; this is what the F-Plan is all about. The F-Plan shows you how to cut your total calorie intake yet at the same time increase your intake of dietary fiber from unrefined cereal foods and the fruits and vegetables that provide it.

When you follow the F-Plan you should:

1. find losing excess pounds to be easier than ever before, because your diet will be considerably more satisfying and filling than any reducing diet you have ever previously tried;

3

2. lose weight *more quickly* than ever before because a larger proportion of the calories you consume will remain undigested, but the important nutrients will be digested;

3. gain all the well-established health advantages of meals high in dietary fiber.

Who says so?

A very large and growing body of scientists engaged in medical and nutrition research throughout the Western world, experts whose reputation is beyond question and who have no cash benefit to gain from their findings.

This is what makes the F-Plan unique.

Not only will you feel more satisfied on less calories, but more of the calories that go into your mouth will, to put it bluntly, go straight through you and down into the toilet. And the less calories from food the body uses, the more it will draw from surplus body fat, adding up to faster weight loss.

Another irresistible appeal to everyone who has tried to reduce: The F-Plan means more weight loss with less demand on willpower!

At the outset we must explain that *dietary fiber* is not the same as *crude fiber*. Until recently only the crude fiber content of plant foods, the tougher outer husks and cell walls, could be measured accurately. Many charts listing the composition of foods still give only the crude fiber content; some product labels list only crude fiber in the ingredients information, and most give no fiber content at all. All along scientists suspected that the *total* fiber in foods of plant origin probably amounted to three or four times as much as crude fiber alone, if only a method could be perfected for measuring the remaining components. Now all that has changed. At last in several laboratories in England and America, top nutritional authorities have been able to assess total dietary fiber in our everyday foods. This recent knowledge enabled us to devise the F-Plan to include popular, familiar, easy-to-prepare foods with outstanding fiber content. That's why the diet is a breakthrough in weight control.

The dietary importance of fiber, or "roughage," as it used to be called, was proclaimed as far back as the 1890s. At that time, in a sanatorium of the Health Reform Institute in Battle Creek, Michigan, a surgeon, Dr. Harvey Kellogg, and an ulcer patient at the clinic, Charles William Post, together invented the first whole-grain breakfast cereals. Health-conscious Americans eagerly bought these new ready-to-serve breakfast cereals, and their modern derivatives still grace breakfast tables all over the U.S.

But most dieticians remained skeptical; because *crude* fiber contained no known nutritive value, why make such a fuss about it? As time went on, to make breakfast cereals more popular with children and a larger segment of the public generally, cereals were refined while vitamins and sugars of various kinds were added. Other cereal foods, including flours, mixes, breads, and pastas, also were heavily refined, until the fiber intake in the American diet dropped to half, or less than half, of what it had been, while total sugar consumption rose from an average of five pounds a year to over a hundred pounds per person a year.

About ten years ago, medical scientists were startled by the observation that many of the "killer" diseases afflicting Western societies were rarely found in less sophisticated communities in the developing world. Why should it be that diseases, such as many forms of cancer, disorders of the bowel, heart disease, and diabetes, which occur frequently here, are almost unknown there? What were these people doing that we weren't doing, and vice versa? One startling answer that emerged was that they were eating foods high in natural fiber while we, in the West, were depriving ourselves of this important material by indulging primarily in softer, easier-to-swallow processed foods.

As evidence of the health benefits of fiber mounted, extolled in best-selling books and popular magazine articles, roughage again became fashionable. Many different cereals high in fiber are available now in all supermarkets, and several kinds of whole-grain breads can be found in all bakery departments.

The original motivation for fiber research was its good-health benefits, along with avoidance of debilitating and often fatal diseases. Then, almost as an accidental byproduct of the research, its benefits in weight reduction began to be observed. Even in Third World countries where food is plentiful, people eating diets high in fiber-rich carbohydrates rarely suffer from that other scourge of Western civilization—obesity. Studies showed that excess weight problems are equally rare among vegetarian high-fiber eaters in America. Why? Was there something in fiber to explain this phenomenon?

As this intriguing observation was verified in repeated surveys, researchers probed into the reasons. Could it be that the calories supplied by a diet high in natural fiber were being digested and absorbed in a different way by the human body? The remarkable answer, revealed by many independently conducted studies, is yes.

In this book you will learn how dietary fiber can be employed to reduce your own weight, and why.

Though a great deal has been written in the last few years about the benefits of dietary fiber as a health factor, somehow the term tends to conjure up an image of being put out to pasture like sheep or cattle. Many have been put off because they think they must add tasteless sawdustlike bran to everything, or that they must give up their favorite pasta dishes, or turn vegetarian. Or they may simply rebel at joining the ranks of health-food enthusiasts.

But how many would guess one can slim down on such high-fiber foods as baked potatoes, chickpeas, whole-wheat macaroni, and sweet corn?

The good news is that dietary fiber is provided by such a wide selection of easily available and delicious foods, you can eat well and pleasantly and at the same time boost fiber intake by between 35 and 50 grams a day—losing weight at the same time.

The F-Plan diet rules are spelled out in detail in Chapter 19. In the chapters that precede it you will find the explanation of why this revolutionary program works, and thus become convinced that the F-Plan is indeed the weight-reducing breakthrough we all have been seeking for so long.

A final point: This diet has nothing to do with the "starch blocker" method of dieting, which physicians and nutritionists frown on. In the F-Plan you can include all those starch foods that are rich in dietary fiber as a basic part of your weight-reducing program, as long as you avoid the refined starches. The fiber in plant foods is nature's own way of controlling your weight.

1

What (and Where) Is Dietary Fiber?

Dietary fiber is a substance obtained from plant foods, as distinct from animal foods. All cereals, fruits, and vegetables contain some dietary fiber, but, just as the calorie content of different foods varies to a great degree, so does the fiber content of different plant foods. Some are excellent sources, while the quantity contained in an average serving of others is negligible. With cereal-based foods, fiber value depends to a large degree on how much has been stripped away in the milling and refining processes. Fruits and vegetables differ so much even in their raw, unprocessed state that you certainly can't say that all of them are useful sources of fiber.

But precisely what is dietary fiber? Well, it could be loosely defined as the cell-wall material of plants—but only loosely, because it also consists of complex substances associated with these cell walls. Dietary fiber can also be described as the carbohydrate material in plant foods (mainly derived from the cell walls) that is not digested by man. Note that phrase "not digested by man," because it gives you your first clue to the slimming advantages of dietary fiber. Food that is not digested cannot be used to provide body fat or calories!

All plants and animals, ourselves included, are made up of cells, but the cell walls of plants are of a more rigid structure. This performs the functions of enclosing cell contents, trapping water, stiffening the plant, and conducting sap. It is tempting to think of dietary fiber as the tough stuff that holds the plant together, and this is true to a degree, but it can be misleading when it comes to locating high-fiber plants by guesswork. Cell walls are made up of a variety of substances, of which only one, cellulose, is truly fibrous in the sense of being filamentous or thread-like.

If you were to take a guess at selecting a high-fiber vegetable you might think of something like celery, which seems to reveal its fiber content unmistakably. Yet peas, extolled by advertisers for their tenderness, in fact contain more than four times the fiber of celery, weight for weight.

Generally, however, high-fiber foods do require more chewing, which gives them yet another advantage, as you will learn later in this book.

Unless you have been living on another planet for the past few years, you have heard that pure wheat bran is the foodstuff with the highest percentage of dietary fiber. This is correct—judged percentage-wise. It is in fact half fiber: 40 to 50 percent. Bran is a byproduct of the milling process used to refine flour. It is largely because the bran is stripped altogether from white flour, and because similar cell-wall material is taken from sugar cane and sugar beets, that our Western diet has become so low in natural fiber content. White flour, the basis of so many of our everyday foods, is fiber-depleted; the finer and softer it is, the more it has been deprived of this important element. Sugar, too, has been totally divested of fiber.

However, the F-Plan does not suggest you obtain your dietary fiber from bran alone, and for some very good reasons. For one thing, bran is a bulky substance, quite unpalatable by itself, and it is not easy to consume more than half an ounce a day. Much more important is the fact that you cannot obtain the full benefit of dietary fiber from bran alone; it must be obtained from a wide range of cereal foods, fruit, and vegetables, to get full health value and the greatest benefit in weight control. Dietary fiber differs from plant to plant. It is a very complex substance and there is still much to be learned about it. Indications are that different forms of fiber may perform different beneficial functions.

The old idea that you could get all necessary fiber simply by adding bran to this and that has been disproved by recent research. Bran helps, by replacing an important element taken out in the refining process, but it provides only part of the dietary fiber needed.

Fresh fruit, for instance, is a rich source of another element in dietary fiber: pectin. Pectin is now recognized as having value in slowing down the digestion and absorption of sugars and fats. Dr. David Jenkins, associate professor of nutritional science at the University of Toronto, describes it as a "sponge" that soaks up glucose (sugar) and fat, slowing the rate of absorption into the bloodstream.

Only recently have researchers in several countries observed and verified that this nonnutritive substance can be a real help to some diabetics—and an aid to dieters.

Researchers in Italy first observed pectin's role in aiding diabetics; since then this benefit has been verified by nutritional scientists in France, Israel, Czechoslovakia, Britain, and the United States. Results have indicated that diabetics need less insulin when given doses of pectin. (While pectin is being prescribed for specific health problems, it should not be taken in its pure form except under a doctor's supervision.)

The many benefits of dietary fiber are still being investigated, and we can expect to learn more of its composition and role in the digestive process as time goes on. Meantime, it is clear that *everyone* needs nonnutritive dietary fiber daily just as much as the nutritive proteins, vitamins, and minerals that are essential elements in our diets. Dietary fiber provides the balance nature devised for the digestive and elimination process; but it should be consumed in natural form, not in pills or extracts.

Even though most people are aware that bran and whole-grain cereal products are excellent sources of fiber, what has been lacking is an up-to-date and down-to-earth guideline for selecting a wide range of high-fiber foods for everyday menus, listed in terms of normal serving portions. Textbooks and scientific reference guides to food composition available in libraries list the components of virtually everything edible, but some give no fiber content at all; others give only crude fiber in percentages. As was already pointed out, this is only part of the story and can be very misleading.

For example, consider watercress. In food component tables it is shown to have 3.3 percent dietary fiber, a higher percentage than an apple, which has only 1.5 percent fiber. You might think therefore that watercress is a very good source. But a reasonably generous portion of watercress, 10 sprigs, provides only 0.5 gram of fiber, because it is so lightweight. By contrast, an average-sized apple, listed as having only 1.5 percent, actually provides 3 to 4 grams of fiber, because it weighs so much more. Carrots have 3.0 percent fiber, but an average portion (½ cup) provides 3.4 grams also.

The best sources of all for those wanting to lose weight are high-fiber foods that tend to be consumed in reasonably large quantities, yet are not excessively high in calories.

A good example is chickpeas (also called garbanzos). These have become very popular both as a salad ingredient and in main-course entrees. A single cup of canned chickpeas, a generous serving for lunch or dinner, contributes 12 grams of fiber, nearly half the quantity of fiber the average American now consumes in an entire day.

Canned baked beans, the kind that come ready to heat and serve, are one of the very top sources of fiber: One cup (an 8-ounce can or half a 16-ounce can) provides 16 grams.

At the other end of the scale, one of the poorer vegetable sources of fiber is cucumber, which contains only 0.4 percent of dietary fiber and tends to be consumed in modest servings. It has a low fiber content and a low portion weight, so its fiber contribution to the average diet is negligible.

Taking this essential "how much is normally eaten" factor into account, we have, with the kind assistance of Derek Miller of London University's Department of Nutrition, compiled the tables starting on page 61.* These, we believe, give the first truly realistic and helpful guide to the fiber content of foods. The tables, based on average portions, show you the whole range of plant foods, from those that are enormously helpful to those that are virtually useless in boosting the fiber content of your diet.

* Dr. James W. Anderson of the Veterans Administration Medical Center in Lexington, Kentucky, was most helpful in providing information on dietary fiber in foods popular with Americans.

2

The Vital Calorie Factor

By including sufficient high-fiber foods in your diet you will actually help your body to shed surplus fat. But this doesn't mean that you can forget about calories. The strength of the F-Plan lies in the way it limits the calories you consume.

Never let anyone, or any diet, convince you that calories don't count in achieving weight loss. They do. They are what reducing is all about.

Calories are units of energy, the energy we need to keep going. We consume these calories in the form of food and use them up in maintaining the body's functions and movements. All foods supply calories, but in widely varying quantities on an ounce-for-ounce basis.

Sometimes—often, in fact—in the Western world, people consume more calories than they need to fuel the body with energy. A percentage of these surplus calories is then stored as body fat, and this is what makes people overweight.

The only way to reverse this situation and become slim again is to supply the body with less calories than it needs for its daily energy requirements, so that it has to draw on the emergency store of calories in its own fat. When you are trying to lose weight you are really eating your own body—eating away the part of it you don't want, that surplus fat! Apart from becoming highly energetic and making the body burn up many more calories daily—a possible but usually very slow method of shedding weight—there is no other way of losing weight than by depriving the body of calories.

All reducing diets that can possibly work are based on

13

calorie reduction, but it is easy to see why people become confused about this. So many diets appear to have no connection with calories.

An example is the once highly popular low-carbohydrate method of weight loss. Dieters were told that they only had to ration carbohydrates, and then they could eat as much as they liked of other foods. These diets are now frowned upon by many medical experts because of their low fiber content. However, it is true that many people succeeded in losing weight on these diets. (These diets could be said to have been half right, in that they cut out refined carbohydrates, but unfortunately without adding fiber-rich carbohydrate foods, which we now know to be of such help.)

The reason for weight loss, though, was calorie reduction. Because so many people in the West eat such a large proportion of their daily calories in the form of refined sugary and starchy foods, when these foods were strictly rationed daily calorie intake usually automatically dropped sufficiently to achieve weight loss. Although people were allowed to eat other foods freely, when they were deprived of their refined carbohydrates they tended not to increase their intake of these alternative foods very much—not enough to make up for the calories they were saving.

Then there are those modern diets that tell you to ration only fats. Fats supply the most calories of all, very many more, weight for weight, than all other foods. All high-calorie foods are fatty, and all high-calorie meals are fatty. So by rationing these foods you cut calorie intake. You are on a low-calorie diet. But since the foods allowed are still refined foods, the fiber content may not be high enough to meet present recommended levels.

Ah, but what about those remarkable diet formulas that say you can eat all you like of a particular food, such as chicken, or steak, or yogurt, as long as you eat only this food or combination of foods? You may have actually heard people raving about the weight losses they attribute to these magical foods. Poor souls, all they were doing was cutting calorie intake—the hard way. You could say their success was based on the "throw-up factor." There is a limit to the quantity of any one particular food you can eat, and continue to eat without other foods, before beginning to feel bored with it and then almost sick at the thought of it.

More scientifically, variety has been found to be a factor in influencing the quantity of food we desire. It is partly because our Western diets are varied (and healthily so, because this ensures a wide range of necessary vitamins and minerals) that we are tempted to overeat. It's amazing how easy and tempting it is to eat a little more when we are offered food of a different flavor and texture—dessert after a very filling meal, for instance. Interestingly enough, even hens and rats have been found to consume more calories when they are offered a varied diet than when they are fed "the same old thing" all the time.

People eating "the same old thing" eat less calories. Restrict a person to any one food, and even if that food is chocolate he or she will almost certainly lose weight. But these diets are, by their nature, eventually self-defeating. After a certain time the very sight of the food allowed becomes off-putting and even repellent. Many people have experience of this from gorging sessions in childhood. My own son, as a small boy, allowed to graze freely on a strawberry field during a "pick your own" expedition and aware that he, unlike our basket, would not be weighed and charged, once achieved a mammoth strawberry-eating feat. That was five years ago, and he hasn't been able to face a strawberry since!

So *all* diets, even those that come complete with generally useless injections and pills, achieve weight loss only by reducing calorie intake.

The F-Plan also reduces your calorie intake in order to allow you to lose weight at sufficient speed. The radical difference between this diet and previous dieting methods is that it makes the food you consume more filling and also renders some of the calories it supplies nonfattening, as you will learn in the next chapter.

3

The Calorie-Fiber Connection

The most dramatic thing about the recent dietary fiber research is that it has, to a degree, altered the basis on which experts have been calculating potential weight loss over the past half century or so—the period during which overweight people have been begging diet doctors and dieticians to help them shed surplus fat.

It is never possible to predict weight loss precisely, even for people on the same diet. This will vary from person to person depending on many individual factors, including the amount of excess weight (the heavier you are, the faster you tend to lose weight) and the degree of energy expended in physical activity. Nevertheless, there is a simple weight-loss equation on which it was possible to estimate the maximum amount of weight likely to be lost each week on any specific calorie allowance. This is based on the difference between the number of calories consumed in food and the number of calories required to keep the body going.

Let us assume that you are a woman of medium height, doing a job like housework, which requires a moderate amount of physical activity, and that you are ten to fifteen pounds overweight and just about to embark on trying to lose it. In these circumstances, it could be roughly assumed that you would be burning up around 2,000 calories a day.

If we were to put you on a reducing diet providing you with 1,500 calories a day, you would be 500 calories short of your requirement, and these would have to be taken from your body fat. It has been scientifically estimated that a pound of your own body fat provides approximately 3,500 calories. So during a week you would be likely to shed one pound of surplus fat.

Obviously, if you followed a stricter diet allowing only 1,000 calories a day, you would draw an additional 500 calories a day from your body fat. With a daily deficit of 1,000 calories you could expect to lose around two pounds a week.

As you see, expected rate of fat loss has always been estimated simply by counting the calories consumed in the form of food, any food, and subtracting them from the number the body requires for energy.

The recent findings about fiber introduce a new factor into this weight-loss equation.

As we have already pointed out, when people eat high-fiber diets they excrete more calories in their stools (feces). In several experiments, scientists have undertaken the task of analyzing the stools of those following high-fiber diets and have found that the calories excreted are measurably greater in number than the calories excreted by those on the normal, varied Western diets, rich in refined carbohydrate foods. Tests indicate that the increased calorie content of the feces amounts to nearly 10 percent when people follow high-fiber diets.

Obviously, those calories that are being flushed away are not being used by the body—which means that the body is having to use more of its own surplus fat to make up for them. So on a 1,000-calorie high-fiber diet the body is going to lose weight more quickly than on a normal 1,000-calorie diet of varied food—or on any other 1,000-calorie diet.

Weight loss depends on the number and *the source* of calories consumed. The rate of weight loss will be influenced not only by the quantity you eat, in terms of calories, but also by which foods you choose to make up that calorie intake.

This is just one of the advantages you gain from high-fiber dieting when you follow the F-Plan slimming method. The benefit of this revolutionary method is based on a whole range of advantages over other reducing diets that add up to faster, easier, more effective weight loss. From the moment you put fiber-rich food into your mouth it starts to give both physical and psychological advantages in filling you, satisfying you, protecting you from feeling hungry again soon, and speeding your weight loss.

The slimming benefits of the F-Plan diet start in the mouth, continue in the stomach, extend to the blood, and reach a grand finale with that final flush!

So let's start with the first mouthful and work our way down the whole digestive tract, to explain fully the marvelous benefits of this new weight-loss method.

4

How Fiber Helps—in Your Mouth

Even before the foods that are rich in dietary fiber start to pass down your throat, they perform a multiplicity of functions that help to reduce the quantity of food you want to eat, and they start to send helpful satiety signals to the brain. A whole range of slimming benefits, both physiological and psychological, come into play right there in your mouth.

One of these benefits is in slowing down your eating. This may not, at first glance, seem to be a major factor, but many experts consider it to be a crucial element in weight control. The rate at which you eat not only strongly influences how much you want to eat but—more surprisingly—it influences the length of time elapsing before you feel the desire to eat again. One of the most fascinating scientific experiments of recent years showed that when people ate meals at a rapid rate they became hungry again more quickly than when they ate precisely the same size meal at a slower rate. Why this happens isn't fully understood, but it is well endorsed by general observation.

Never underestimate the role of eating speed in slimming and weight control. It is much more important than most people realize. If a group of people sitting at a dining table had their entire bodies shrouded under some tentlike garment, there are two ways by which the expert observer of eating behavior could differentiate the fat from the slim. One of the things the expert would note would be that, however big the meal—and let us assume that overlarge portions were served—some people would consume every morsel and leave an entirely clean plate. These would almost certainly be the overweight people. This is something you can observe for yourself in almost any restaurant.

Overweight people, particularly the heavily overweight, rarely stop eating until they have finished everything on the plate. Slim people, in contrast, usually stop when they feel satisfied. In the case of an overlarge meal this would mean that the slim people would put down their knives and forks and leave some food.

Overweight people seem to lack a "stop mechanism." This appears to be one of their basic problems. Effortlessly slim people are governed by their body's requirement for food and are bullied by messages from the body—"That's it, I've had enough"—at the appropriate time. "Honestly," slim people say, "I couldn't eat another morsel." And they really mean it.

In contrast, overweight people seem to get much less strong and effective stop signals from the body, and this is largely because of the other factor, the major clue, that our eating-behavior expert would be using in his or her "guess who's overweight" game.

The overweight people would eat more rapidly than the slim people, as has been shown in several scientific experiments. A recent experiment in America showed that people of normal weight might start eating at a reasonably rapid pace at the beginning of a meal, when their hunger is at a peak, but this eating rate will steadily slow down as the meal progresses. The overweight people in this experiment, however, kept eating at the same fast pace throughout the meal.

Again, this is something you can observe for yourself in any public eating place. Overweight people tend to eat in a nonstop motion. As one mouthful of food is being chewed, another is on the fork and on its way up—ready to be put in the mouth the second that the first mouthful starts on its way down the throat.

From my own observations, generally the greater the weight problem, the faster the rate of eating. Once I sat with a psychiatrist, a specialist in eating behavior, and observed a hugely overweight couple (quite unaware that we were watching them) eating their restaurant breakfasts. The quantity of food collected from the help-yourself buffet was enormous, and the speed with which it was consumed was almost supersonic. The husband not only forked food into his mouth with an almost nonstop movement of his right hand, he also held a corn muffin in his left hand so that he could keep eating during the time it took to reload his fork. Chewing must have been absolutely minimal. Needless to say, silence prevailed throughout the meal. And at the end of it, after eating what must have been at least half a dozen scrambled eggs, plus bacon, sausages, and several rolls, the couple got up to reload their plates.

This is an extreme example, but most of us who have any kind of weight problem, however small, can benefit from slowing down our eating, for some very sound scientific reasons.

After food is put into the mouth it takes a few minutes (usually around five) for it even to start having any physical effect in satisfying the hungry body. At a fast eating pace and with a minimum amount of chewing—and very little chewing is usually required with refined sugary and starchy foods—an awful lot of calories can be consumed in five minutes.

As eating time continues, the body sends out more and more satiety signals, but it is estimated that it takes about twenty minutes for a meal to have its full effect in filling our stomachs and sending out all the other physical signals of sufficiency. That is why speedy eaters, who eat their fill in perhaps ten or fifteen minutes, often feel overfull some minutes after the meal. Most of us, the slim as well as the overweight, have uttered that plaintive wail: "Oh, I shouldn't have done it!" as we patted our far from comfortable stomachs after a particularly tempting feast, like Christmas dinner.

"Slow down your eating" is excellent classic advice for those with a weight problem—and many of those who have struggled long in the battle of the bulge have probably read it before, and even tried to follow it. Quite probably they failed, or gave up trying after a time.

Why? Because the rate of eating is a deeply established habit, and all deeply established habits are very difficult to break. If you were advised to speak more slowly it would probably take months of effort, repeated conscious effort, before you succeeded in altering the speed at which you spoke. The same would apply to changing your accent. Think of the effort that Professor Higgins had to put in with Eliza!

Slowing down a habitual eating rate isn't easy and tends to need prolonged effort—and this is where a high-fiber diet starts to have its first effect in helping you to eat less. It automatically slows down the rate of eating for you! And for a number of reasons, not just one.

First of all, unprocessed plant foods tend to be bulky. You get a large volume or bulk of food for a small or moderate number of calories, and that in itself is going to necessitate considerably more chewing and take considerably more time. Take sugar and apples for comparison. The average American consumes at least five ounces of sugar in a day. In the way it is grown and gathered, in cane or beet, sugar contains an appreciable content of dietary fiber, but this is stripped away completely in the refining process to leave no fiber at all in the sugar we buy in packets or consume in cakes, cookies, alcoholic mixed drinks or other drinks, and nearly all processed foods.

Many people consume a good deal of sugar in drinks. It takes hardly any time at all to swoosh down a can of cola, and neither does this seem to have any effect in satisfying the appetite. Most people find it easy to drink large quantities of caloric drinks, sweet or alcoholic, without in any way lessening or delaying their appetite for the next meal—and these drinks, and sugar itself, are perhaps the ultimate example of fiber-free calories. By consuming calories without any dietary fiber at all, you can down a very large number of calories, at a very fast rate, with very little effect in satisfying the appetite.

And when refined sugar is combined with refined flour to make cake or desserts, the chewing required tends to be minimal.

It is somewhat unrealistic to imagine people gnawing away at sugar cane or sugar beet, so as an example at the opposite extreme let us consider apples. Apples, though a useful source of vitamins and mineral, are mostly water, sugar (fructose), and fiber (which includes pectin). Only the sugar supplies calories. But the amount of sugar in each apple is so low that to consume 5 ounces would require eating at least a dozen apples. You can imagine how long that would take—and how filling all those apples would be. If the dietary fiber were removed, the apple would become apple juice. This way, those apple sugar calories could be consumed very quickly without the appetite-satisfying effect. So it is the dietary fiber that has the slowing-down and filling-up effect.

This principle is true of all foods. Dietary fiber has the

general effect of filling you up, slowing down eating, and satisfying the appetite in this and many other ways.

But this isn't the only way in which dietary fiber slows down eating. The texture as well as the bulk of fiber-rich foods helps to put on the brakes.

The pleasure of eating is largely the pleasure of taste. In natural fiber-rich foods the taste-evoking substances appear to remain intact within the cell walls, which have not been stripped away by refining processes. Therefore, the taste of an unprocessed food is not fully appreciated unless it is chewed. This may be one reason why fiber-rich foods are normally automatically chewed more thoroughly than processed foods.

There is yet another reason why many fiber-rich foods slow down eating and add to satisfaction. Food is not swallowed with comfort unless, or until, it is soft and moist. If it is dry and unyielding we automatically chew it until it becomes comfortable to swallow. Many high-fiber fruits and vegetables, nuts, and dry breakfast cereals (shredded wheat, for instance, as opposed to porridge) need a good deal of chewing before they can be comfortably swallowed. Cooking, particularly boiling, reduces but does not wholly remove the firmness of food.

Scientists have done careful experiments to confirm the benefits of dietary fiber in slowing down eating. Sensibly comparing two foods of a very similar nature, they monitored a group of people eating a meal consisting entirely of whole-wheat bread, which contains 8.5 percent dietary fiber, and compared them with a group eating a meal of white bread, which contains only 2.7 percent dietary fiber. The whole-wheat bread took 11 minutes longer to consume (45 minutes) than the white bread (34 minutes).

Dietary fiber means that a food requires more chewing

and also more swallowing. During prolonged chewing, more saliva is secreted, and this adds to the volume of the food in the mouth. That obviously necessitates more swallowing. Although it takes a few minutes for the body to send out any strong signals of satiety, it is probable that chewing and swallowing do begin to send messages to the brain.

Nearly all of us, the overweight as well as the slim, have some body controls that limit our eating capacity. Otherwise, some people would indeed quite literally eat themselves to death. (In fact, during the past year there were cases of disturbed people doing just that.) The vast majority of people have built-in controls, and these seem to differ in the overweight and the slim only in their degree of effectiveness. The major control mechanisms appear to be the state of fullness of the stomach, a satiety system in the brain known as the appestat, and, according to some experts, blood sugar.

In experiments with rats, increased electrical activity was recorded in the satiety area of the brain during chewing and swallowing. This indicates that chewing and swallowing at least start to bring our bodily eating controls into action by sending the first satiety signals to the brain—and that the more chewing and swallowing we do, the more effective this is likely to be.

So far we have dealt only with the physical benefits of fiber-rich foods in the mouth. The psychological benefits might well be just as great.

Chewing gives psychological satisfaction, and in scientific experiments gum chewing has been found to help reduce tension. Psychiatrists working in the area of weight control have discovered that we need our "psychological fill" as well as our physical fill of food in order to feel content with what we have eaten.

It has been found that when someone eats a snack while mentally absorbed in other things—perhaps a mother grabbing her own meal in between attempts to coax food down a baby, or a viewer eating a TV snack while totally involved in the latest plots of "Dallas"—the food has little effect in satisfying hunger. Often, for instance, after the baby has been put to sleep the mother will sit down and eat another meal.

We seem to need to get a sufficient daily quota of conscious relaxation and pleasure from our food, and obviously this occurs while the food is in the mouth. Little wonder that a meal of mainly refined foods, gulped down in seconds, tends to lead to second helpings to extend the time of eating, or another meal or snack shortly afterward to "bulk out" the eating pleasure of the day.

In this chapter you have discovered many ways in which foods containing dietary fiber can make you feel more satisfied—and the food has not yet gone down the throat. See what happens when high-fiber food reaches the stomach.

5

How Fiber Fills Your Stomach—and for Longer

Dietary fiber is a spongelike material that absorbs and holds water as it is chewed in the mouth and passes down the gastrointestinal tract. This means that fiber-rich foods swell to a greater bulk, to fill the stomach, than any other foods.

The state of fullness of the stomach is obviously going to influence your appetite. A derivative of cellulose has long been used as a diet aid for this reason. Cellulose is one of the substances present in dietary fiber.

Many of the pills and capsules that are sold as appetite suppressants consist largely of methyl cellulose. The only problem is that you can't get enough of this material in pills and capsules to provide enough bulk to have any realistically helpful effect in filling the stomach.

However, when scientists Derek Miller and Dr. Elizabeth Evans conducted tests at London University, adding 20 grams of cellulose to people's daily diets, they found this did indeed automatically reduce calorie intake. Overweight people consumed less calories without even trying to do so. So a sufficient quantity of cellulose—and on the F-Plan you get plenty—does help you to eat less.

This large bulk of material in the stomach is just one of the factors that make you feel more satisfied on less food. Equally important is the fact that fiber-rich food stays in the stomach longer than fiber-depleted food. The gastric acids have a much tougher job to do when they have to fight their way through fibrous cell-wall material. This produces two results—both beneficial in weight loss. Food in a fiber-rich diet stays in the stomach longer; and it seems probable that the food is less efficiently digested as it goes through the digestive tract.

The second factor is less obviously helpful at first glance—but what it adds up to is calorie saving!

The cell walls themselves are totally indigestible and do not provide calories. This factor is taken into account in giving the calorie values of carbohydrate foods. However, it seems highly likely that some of the calorie-supplying substances associated with the cell walls are not digested either when a diet is high in natural fiber. This would help to account for some of the extra calories expelled in the feces of those consuming fiber-rich foods.

So when you eat your F-Plan fiber-rich diet you get a greater and more filling bulk of food in the stomach, the food stays there longer, and it is likely that less of those potentially fat-producing calories are digested.

Yet another advantage is the prevention of stomach discomfort, often the trigger for diet-breaking snacks. Unless stomach acids have a job to do in digesting food, they tend to cause discomfort, and dieters often find themselves turning to extra food to quell the unpleasant acidic feeling they get when the stomach is largely empty. Fiber-rich foods keep the stomach acids under control for long periods because those acids have to work longer and harder at digestion processes.

It is only when the fiber-rich food leaves the stomach that it starts passing through the body at a faster pace, giving the well-documented health benefits. It stays longer where you need it to stay—in the stomach—and moves more swiftly where you need it to move more swiftly, through the intestine and bowel.

But we are far from being at the end of the chain of slimming benefits that are achieved by a diet rich in natural fiber. There is the blood factor, too, which can also provide a major benefit, as you will learn in the next chapter.

6

Rebound Hunger—How Fiber Beats It

One of the major problems that gave carbohydrate foods in general the reputation of being fattening would be described by doctors as "rebound hypoglycemia." The rest of us might put the same thing in much more simple terms by voicing that popular complaint, "When you've eaten a Chinese meal you feel hungry again in a couple of hours." This kind of comment might well follow a Chinese meal consisting largely of white processed rice. Carbohydrate foods—it used to be thought all carbohydrate foods—do indeed have a tendency to produce a rebound hunger. There is a scientific explanation.

One of the purposes of digestion is to reduce food to a substance that can be absorbed in the bloodstream as sugar. Blood sugar needs to be kept up to the correct level in order to allow both body and mind to function correctly, and the body is very clever at informing us of its requirements. When blood sugar drops below the required level the body sends out signals that are often interpreted by the mind as "I am feeling hungry." Blood sugar level is one of the physical factors in determining the state of hunger. Generally, when the blood sugar level is high, we don't feel hungry—when it is low, we do.

All carbohydrates, sugars, and starches are converted into blood sugar. The only difference is that sugars and starches in refined carbohydrate foods are more quickly converted into blood sugar. After a meal consisting largely of refined carbohydrate food the blood sugar level goes up very quickly, which would seem to be a good thing in satisfying the appetite. But then comes the snag.

The body has to have control mechanisms to regulate all its functions—mechanisms to excrete an appropriate quantity of the water we drink, for instance; otherwise, since we tend to drink so much more than we require, we would eventually burst. Similarly, we have mechanisms to excrete most of the excess salt that we eat, since most of us consume more than ten times the amount necessary for our bodily needs.

Blood sugar level goes up on the digestion of food. But if it were to go up and up and up the blood would become absolutely saturated with sugar, which would do us no good at all. Therefore, we have a control mechanism to bring down the blood sugar level when it begins to reach unhealthy peaks. This control mechanism involves the substance called insulin, secreted by the pancreas.

When the blood sugar level shoots up rapidly, the pancreas hurries into action and secretes a large quantity of insulin to keep the situation under control. Insulin in the bloodstream reduces the quantity of blood sugar by helping the blood sugar to be used by cells. All is well for an hour or so. But after about two hours the excess amount of insulin in the blood tends to have an effect that isn't at all helpful to the person seeking to control hunger and food intake. It suppresses the blood sugar level—not just back to the level before the meal, but to even lower than the pre-meal level.

This is what is known as rebound hypoglycemia. On the basis of this scientific fact you can readily understand why many doctors have for years discouraged overweight people from eating carbohydrate-rich foods. However, during all those years of "cut your carbohydrates" advice, which impressed itself so much on the public that many people are still overwhelmed with guilt at the sight of a slice of bread or a potato, all high-carbohydrate foods were grouped together as culprits in causing this rebound hunger that led to excessive eating.

More recent research has shown that it is only some carbohydrate foods that cause this problem, not all of them. No prizes for guessing that it is the refined sugary and starchy foods that cause this rebound hunger, and natural fiber-rich foods that do not. The latter are more slowly converted into blood sugar, mainly because of the digestive processes described in the previous chapter. This may well be the reason why the rebound hunger problem does not arise when carbohydrate foods are consumed in their natural fiber-rich form. Whatever the reason, repeated tests have shown that the inclusion of sufficient dietary fiber in meals prevents the excessive output of insulin that so often leads to hunger and snack-eating on diets in which the carbohydrates are processed and refined—yet another reason why dietary fiber helps to control your hunger and your weight.

7

The Fiber Calorie Saving

Once the residue of a meal rich in natural fiber leaves the stomach after its lengthy residence there, it speeds down the intestine at a faster pace. In doing so it saves the dieter from the common curse of constipation, which frequently accompanies other reducing diets. Medical research that you will read about later in this book indicates that this faster and more efficient transit may well be helpful in preventing many much more serious illnesses of the lower intestine and bowel, including cancer.

When the feces are finally expelled, many studies have shown, this waste matter has a higher calorie content than that excreted by people following a normal Western diet containing refined carbohydrates.

Happily for most of us, who are inclined to overeat occasionally or frequently, all the calories consumed in food are not used by the body for energy or fat storage. There is a natural wastage of at least 5 percent on any diet. But tests so far have clearly shown that dietary fiber increases the wastage and indicated that generally, the higher the fiber content, the higher the wastage of calories.

In one scientific experiment it was found that a daily increase of 10 grams of dietary fiber, by the addition of more fruit, vegetable, and whole-wheat bread to an ordinary Western diet, increased the number of calories excreted in a bowel movement by nearly 90. With still more additional dietary fiber, 32 grams a day, the stools were found to contain 210 calories on average. However, it must be added that these subjects were consuming quite a large quantity of food and were not attempting to lose weight.

Just why there are more calories in the human excreta following the intake of a high-fiber diet is less than fully understood at the present stage of scientific research. One source of these surplus calories excreted is obviously the nondigestible cell-wall material that forms much of the dietary fiber itself. This is taken into account when calorie figures are given for carbohydrate foods.

Scientific calorie charts frequently speak of "available carbohydrate calories." This means that the nondigestible calories in the plant cell walls, which will eventually be expelled in the feces, have already been subtracted in order to give a realistic calorie figure for each carbohydrate food. However, there are other, additional calories in the feces expelled after high-fiber eating, in the form of fat and protein. These are not accounted for in the calorie figures. Nor are they fully explained—although less efficient digestion in general is probably a reasonably accurate explanation.

But we have dwelled long enough on this final stage of the fiber slimming story. Suffice it to say that if you are cutting calories in order to lose weight at a speedy pace, every calorie counts—every calorie that you don't make available to your body!

By following a normal mixed 1,000-calorie diet of protein, fat, and refined carbohydrate foods you will be making most of those calories available to your body. But you will still lose weight at a good pace. By concentrating on including a greater percentage of high-fiber vegetables, fruits, and cereal foods in your diet you will be making less of those 1,000 calories available to your body. So you should lose weight at an even faster rate.

The dual aim of most dieters is to become slimmer and fitter by following a diet. No one wants to be slim and ill. These days the principal dietary health recommendations of all major nutritional bodies in the Western world are: Eat less fat, less sugar, and more dietary fiber. That is precisely what you will do on the F-Plan. Later in the book we discuss the health benefits of the F-Plan in detail. But now for your guide to losing weight the easy, speedy way—on the F-Plan.

8

Calories: How Low Can You Go?

Hunger is a problem that simply should not arise on the F-Plan, even though you are restricting the actual number of calories consumed each day. This does not mean that you cannot possibly be tempted by the sight of a chocolate bar or the aroma of a steak or a hamburger, but you will more easily be able to resist. Because the calories consumed are in the form of particularly bulky, filling, and satisfying food, your appetite will not be sharpened nor your willpower lowered by actual physical hunger.

We live in a world where food temptations flaunt themselves all around us. They pop up in the commercials on the TV screen, at popcorn stands at the movies, at gourmet food shops, and in bakery windows. In the Western world it is almost impossible to be far from the sight of food. Even if shipwrecked, you would probably be rescued by a passing cruise ship, on which you would be stuffed endlessly with food to compensate for the boredom of the interminable view of the sea. Food, in our society, is used for many reasons other than simply to satisfy hunger. It is used for comfort, pleasure, socializing, celebrating, time-filling, seduction—to name just a few of the alternatives.

Obviously, the person who is not actually hungry is considerably less vulnerable to the temptations of our food-filled Western world. Psychiatrists studying shopping behavior have found—not surprisingly—that the hungry woman is much more inclined to succumb to impulse food buys. She generally fills her supermarket cart more fully when she shops just before a meal than if she shops shortly after one, when her hunger is fully satisfied. Supermarket managers, always seeking new ways to cram more food down us, would be wise to offer a special shop-before-lunch discount!

When you are eating a fiber-rich diet there are restraining limits on how many calories you can actually manage to consume in a day—even if you aren't trying to lose weight. This was illustrated most illuminatingly by a recent study in which a group of people were asked to eat more than a pound of potatoes each day (baked in their skins, not fried) in addition to whatever other food they could manage to eat. By adding these potatoes, a bulky food of reasonably high-fiber content, they actually lost some weight over a three-month period! The potatoes were so filling that there wasn't a great deal of room left for all the other foods they usually ate. The same remarkable result occurred in a similar experiment in which people were asked to consume a generous quantity of whole-grain bread each day. Again they lost weight without attempting to do so.

This was impressive. But it certainly wouldn't be fair to claim that all anyone need do in order to shed surplus weight is to add sufficient fiber-rich foods to the diet—or switch from refined-carbohydrate foods to natural fiber-rich foods like whole-grain breads. Though weight loss might well result, as the experiments show, it would tend to be very slow.

In the future, when you have become slim, the change from refined-carbohydrate foods to their high-fiber alternatives should be sufficient to keep you that way. Certainly it will do so if you also put some restraints on your intake of fats. This is clearly indicated by the slenderness of those in the Third World societies who live on plentiful supplies of foods high in fiber content. So the F-Plan does have a great stay-slim bonus. Food preferences are very much dictated by habit, and those who get into the habit of choosing the fiber-rich foods gradually come to prefer them.

However, most people aiming to shed surplus weight are also aiming to do so reasonably swiftly. To be frank, the basic aim of most dieters is to lose two tons by yesterday! This attitude is undertandable, and slimming experts who drearily continue to tell us to "be satisfied just to lose weight slowly: half a pound a week is enough" have little or no understanding of human psychology.

The F-Plan requires less actual effort than any other slimming diet you have followed before. But all slimming diets—the F-Plan included—require some degree of conscious effort and self-control. In order to sustain effort, in this and all other areas of life, we need the feedback of reward—ideally, short-term reward rather than some far-distant pot of gold, way off at the end of the rainbow. The essential reward for the dieter is that weekly weight loss. There are few joys in life to compare with that of stepping on the scale and discovering that you weigh measurably less this week than you did last.

A miserable half pound is barely recordable. Any seasoned dieter knows full well that she can cheat that weight off the normal set of bathroom scales by shifting her stance a little or rushing off to empty the bladder, remove the dentures, and so on. Yes, don't think we weren't watching you. . . . A measurable weight loss needs to be at least in the region of two pounds a week in order to provide that reward so essential to sustained effort. You can't cheat off two pounds! In slimming, success tends to breed success. Every manager of a reducing club knows that it is the member who registers a good weight loss at her weekly weigh-in who is most likely to keep up her dieting and return to the club next week, while the member who records a disappointingly low weight loss is the most likely to drop out. In dieting, failure does not make us try harder. Usually, it makes us give up.

On the F-Plan we are aiming for an average weekly weight loss in the region of three pounds in order to keep spirits up as weight goes down. The loss could well be considerably higher, particularly if you are male or heavily overweight; but overhigh expectations can be just as demoralizing as very slow weight loss, so we are taking a restrained attitude.

On the F-Plan the calories will be consumed in food that is more filling, and your body will waste more of them than on other slimming diets. However, we recommend that you keep to the usual recommended calorie intakes for weight loss, and reap the additional advantages in ease and speed, rather than try to eat even less calories than usually recommended in a diet. Remember, most dieters fail to stick to it. The F-Plan's extra filling power can most help you by getting you right to slim-weight target. The "easy" diet is the one that succeeds, because it is the one you continue to follow until you are slim.

To shed surplus weight with the F-Plan, allow yourself a maximum of 1,500 calories a day and an absolute minimum of 1,000 calories a day. You may choose to set your daily calorie intake anywhere between those two limits. These recommendations will guide you to your own ideal daily calorie limits for successful weight loss.

Allow Yourself 1,500 Calories Daily

• If you are a male, of at least medium height, and more than seven or eight pounds over desirable weight. Men have a greater daily calorie requirement than women, so they can lose weight on more generous slimming diets and generally record considerably larger weekly weight losses.

This is unfair, but something that even women's liberation cannot change. Few men could fail to lose weight at a satisfactory rate on a daily allowance of 1,500 calories.

• If you are female, more than 30 pounds overweight, and just embarking on a weight-loss program—as opposed to switching from another slimming diet on which you have already lost some of your surplus weight. The more heavily overweight people are, the more swiftly they can shed surplus fat on a slimming diet. This rate of loss tends to slow down as weight goes down and the metabolism adjusts, to some degree, to dieting. So if you are starting out with a good deal of weight to lose, it is wise to allow scope for reducing calorie intake in the later stages of dieting. Start on 1.500 calories daily, and work your way gradually down to 1,000 daily in order to maintain a good, encouraging rate of loss.

Allow Yourself 1,000 Calories Daily

• If you are a small man, with only a few pounds of surplus weight, and are in a big hurry to lose it;
• If you are female and less than fifteen pounds overweight;
• If you are female and more than fifteen pounds overweight, but have already been dieting and have reached a stage at which continued weight loss is becoming more difficult.

Set Your Daily Calorie Intake Between 1,000 and 1,500 (If You Wish) by Taking into Account the Following:

These factors tend to increase speed of weekly weight loss on a diet:

• Being male.
• Being heavily overweight.
• Being at the start of a slimming program, rather than at a midway stage.
• Being in the habit of eating a generous quantity of food—the more you have been eating, the greater the initial weight-loss impact when you switch to a slimming diet.
• Being involved in a job that necessitates a good deal of physical activity (housework, unfortunately, does not rate high in this way), or taking part in a good deal of sport or walking (that ten-minute daily stroll doesn't really rate here, either).

These factors tend to slow speed of weight loss on a diet:

• Being female.
• Being only a few pounds overweight.
• Being at the tail end of a slimming campaign. Those last few pounds can prove the most stubborn, but the F-Plan will help.
• Having a naturally restrained appetite, which probably means that you are only a few pounds overweight and gained this weight over a lengthy period. We all think we eat less than we do!
• Being a sedentary type of person. This doesn't just mean doing a sedentary job but refers rather to the type of person (who could well be a housewife, doing a basically nonsedentary type of job) who calls the children to bring something from the next room rather than getting up herself, or who goes to great lengths to avoid trips up and down stairs, or who will drive around for five minutes to find a parking spot near the exit of the parking lot rather than walk for two minutes. The sum total of all those little movements makes a big difference to daily calorie expen-

diture and varies a good deal among individuals. The people who move a good deal are often described as being "full of nervous energy." It is not the so-called nervous aspect that burns up the calories, but the frequent physical movement. These always-on-the-move people are usually slim.

In determining your slimming calorie intake, remember that it must include all the calories you drink, as well as those you eat. (More about this in Chapter 10.)

9

Fiber: How High Can You Go?

Before 1919, no statistics on intake of dietary fiber were collected or recorded, but from what is known of the way people used to eat, before the days of so many refined flours and processed foods, it is believed that today we consume half as much fiber, or less, as our great-grandparents.

The average modern American is thought to consume around 20 grams daily. In contrast, some African tribes have been found to have a total fiber intake of between 130 and 150 grams a day, while even in the poorest Asian and African countries the intake is between 40 and 60 grams daily. Yet not only are the major killer diseases of the Western world virtually unknown in these high-fiber-consuming societies, so is obesity.

The figures of average fiber consumption include both the highs and the lows, which means some Americans may be consuming no more than 6 to 10 grams of fiber a day. Those who are extremely overweight are more likely to be among the lower consumers of dietary fiber. Studies have indicated that the weight-conscious, brainwashed by years of "cut out those carbohydrates" advice, tend to avoid the bread and potatoes that supply a good deal of the fiber in most people's diets.

Dieting and nutritional fallacies die hard. As you embark on the F-Plan you might have to work quite energetically to convince yourself that the supposed virtues of the old low-carbohydrate method of dieting have been disproved by recent research. Medical experts no longer approve of this low-carbohydrate method of dieting—largely because of the limits it places on the intake of cereals, fruits, and root vegetables. Whole-grain bread and potatoes are no longer considered the baddies in health and obesity. Fats and sugars have revealed themselves as the real villains.

And, when you think about it, did you succeed in getting permanently slim by struggling to cut out carbohydrates for all those years?

When you follow the F-Plan menus you can hardly fail to increase daily dietary fiber intake considerably—even if you don't bother to count the grams.

A daily intake of 20 grams is provided by just two pieces of fruit and our F-Plan granola-type mix called Fiber-Filler (see page 53), which you are required to eat each day as part of this slimming plan. *All* the meals, from which you can choose freely, have been specially devised to contain a good percentage of those foods that supply a significant quantity of dietary fiber.

You will find it easy to consume 35 grams of fiber daily, and we suggest this as the lower limit in order to achieve the slimming benefits described in the previous chapters. Those keeping to a strict 1,000-calories-a-day allowance will usually find this to be a realistic target. Obviously, if you are eating more fiber-rich food, you are likely to eat more grams of fiber. Those allowing themselves 1,500 calories daily might reach a fiber intake of 50 grams daily. We advise this as the higher limit.

All the meals on the F-Plan menu are fiber-counted for you. Don't worry about small day-to-day variations in intake, or aim for precise figures—simply choose your menus to provide between 35 grams and 50 grams of dietary fiber each day.

10

What (and How Much) to Drink

On the F-Plan you are asked to drink a generous amount
of calorie-free liquid, but only a very modest quantity of
calorie-supplying liquid.

One liquid is obligatory. You must have a cup of skim
milk each day. This is to help ensure nutritional balance in
your diet and, in particular, to supply calcium, because
dietary fiber can hinder the absorption of calcium to some
degree. There is no evidence of health problems arising
from this particular factor, but on this healthy diet we
want to take extra care to ensure all essential nutrients.
You will also need to use at least part of this milk with
your cereal breakfasts.

Doctors who prescribe high-fiber diets for health problems sometimes advocate a generous daily intake of fluid.
One of the aims and functions of a high-fiber diet is to
sustain a large bulk of semifluid matter in the stomach and
to produce softer and bulkier feces. The fiber itself will
ensure this, but the extra fluid may help it a little—certainly the fluid has to come from somewhere, and it will
do no harm if it is calorie-free. Calorie-free fluids do not
add to body fat, hinder weight loss, or cause fluid reten-
tion in those of normal health. The idea that they do so is
one of the most persistent slimming myths of all.

Neither, to put another old fallacy to rest, is drinking
with meals "fattening," if the drinks are calorie-free.
Drinking with meals the correct way can actually be slimming, in that it can helpfully add to the time it takes to
consume high-fiber meals. The right way is to put down
knife and fork in order to take a sip of water (or other
calorie-free liquid) after a mouthful of food has been

chewed and swallowed. The wrong or "fattening" way to drink with meals is to use the drink to swill food down the throat before it has been swallowed, because then it will speed rather than slow the ingestion of food.

The reason you are asked to be restrained in drinking caloric drinks is that these, even more than refined carbohydrate foods, have the opposite effect from fiber-rich foods in nearly all those steps in the consumption process that influence your degree of hunger. While fiber-rich foods are chewed slowly, caloric drinks require no chewing at all and go down the throat in a split second. While fiber-rich foods fill the stomach for lengthy periods, calories supplied in fluid alone pass through more quickly than any digested from solid foods.

Observers of eating behavior have noted that people can take in very large numbers of calories in the form of liquids without noticeably diminishing their appetite for food at all.

Please read the following very important instructions about drinking while you are following the F-Plan.

Daily Milk Allowance

Your daily half pint or 1 cup (8 ounces) of skim milk is absolutely essential to the F-Plan. One cup of skim milk provides just 84 calories. Reconstituted nonfat dry milk (available in bulk in all supermarkets) has even less: 80 calories to the 8-ounce cup. As a beverage, cultured buttermilk rates the same, 80 calories to the glass, though of course buttermilk is no good in coffee or tea or over breakfast cereal. The calories in whole milk (Grade A homogenized) total almost twice that of skim milk: 161 in an 8-ounce cup. In between there are other choices: Light One, with 1 percent butterfat, has 110 calories per cup. Light Two, with 2 percent butterfat, has 130 calories.

There is also cultured acidophilus milk, which has 110 calories per 8-ounce cup, but, like buttermilk, this is suitable only as a beverage.

The sample daily menus have been designed to include *skim milk at 84 calories a glass.* If you choose the lower-calorie reconstituted nonfat milk at 80 calories a cup, you can allow an additional 4 calories elsewhere in your daily menu; if you choose one of the more caloric milks, you should adjust the rest of your meals to account for the additional calories you'll get from the milk.

Calorie-free Drinks

There are many drinks to choose from that contain no calories at all, or a negligible quantity. These include tea and coffee (if you add no sugar and the milk is from your daily quota), ice water, either from the tap or bottled spring water, bottled seltzer, mineral waters, and low-calorie carbonated drinks, which include Tab, Diet Pepsi, and Fresca. However, others you may have considered low-calorie aren't really. Bitter lemon contains 192 calories in a 12-ounce bottle; the same size bottle of tonic water has 132 calories. If only one-third of a bottle (4 ounces) is poured over ice, you are still consuming 64 bitter lemon calories and 44 of tonic water.

Fruit Juices

Fruit juices are not allowed on the F-Plan. This is one of the ways in which this new method differs from diets of the past. The reason is that fruit juices are simply fruit stripped of its natural fiber content. When you drink orange juice you are getting all the calories that are present in the orange in the form of sugar, but with none of the fiber-filling power. When you buy a small can of frozen concentrated orange juice you are getting the fiber-free contents of a large quantity of oranges, at a cost of more than 300 calories per can. Many people could easily consume a full can, diluted, during a hot summer day, and it would have little if any effect in reducing an appetite for solid food. To consume the same quantity of calories in the form of whole oranges you would have to eat about five of them. Obviously this would have some realistic effect in satisfying the appetite.

Manufacturers are doing the weight-prone no favor in removing fiber from fruits to make them into juices. Scientific tests recorded a great reduction in satiety level when subjects were fed apple juice (apples with their fiber removed), compared with the same quantity of apples eaten whole. The apple juice speeded the fiber-stripped apple through the mouth and stomach and also raised the blood sugar level in a way that led to the rebound hunger described in a previous chapter. The apples produced both the weight-control benefits of high bulk and a lengthy period in the stomach—and they did not lead to rebound hunger.

By getting used to eating oranges rather than drinking orange juice, eating apples rather than drinking apple juice, and so on, you are establishing a good habit that will help to control your weight in the future.

Fruit-juice production is one of the refining processes that can unfortunately help to increase our intake of calories on a modern Western diet.

Alcohol

As far as health, fitness, and fast weight loss are concerned, it is obviously better to avoid alcohol while following the F-Plan or any other slimming diet.

However, those are all physical factors. There are psychological factors to be taken into account, too. If you feel deprived and miserable by not being allowed an early evening drink, or a glass of wine with your evening meal, it is usually better to allow yourself a little alcohol while dieting. Otherwise it is unlikely that you are going to keep to the diet for very long. However, here is the vital F-Plan rule:

If you are allowing yourself a daily ration of alcohol, allow these calories in addition to a minimum of 1,000 calories' worth of food and milk from the F-Plan menus. First, allow 84 calories from the cup of skim milk, and another 100 calories for your daily apple and orange. Then make up a minimum of 800 calories (more, if you are allowing yourself 1,500 a day) from the Fiber-Filler (see page 53) and the meals on the F-Plan menus. After that you can add the appropriate number of calories from alcohol.

Nearly everyone, female as well as male, can shed surplus fat at a good pace on 1,250 calories a day, and the vast majority of people will achieve a satisfactory weight loss on 1,500 calories a day. So nearly everyone can afford to drink a little alcohol while they are dieting, if they wish.

Alcohol does not provide any useful nutrients or fiber; hence the reason for consuming 1,000 daily calories from food and milk, to ensure good nutrition, before adding any "empty" alcohol calories.

If preferred, calories can be averaged out on a weekly rather than a daily basis. For instance, as long as you average 8,750 calories a week you will shed weight just as quickly by having as many as 1,870 a day on Saturdays and Sundays, and only 1,000 each weekday, as you would by counting precisely 1,250 calories a day for all seven days of the week. This fact can be used to advantage by those who drink alcohol occasionally—perhaps only once or twice a week on social occasions, and not every day.

On the following pages you will find a calorie chart that provides a very realistic way of measuring the calories consumed in the form of alcoholic drinks.

The "If You Must" Alcohol Calorie Chart

Those who decide to include some alcohol in their daily dieting calorie allowance will find their honest and realistic guide to calories here. We say "honest" because a great deal of self-deception goes on in counting calories from drinks during dieting. Bar measures can usually be relied upon for accuracy. Home measures rarely can. It is so easy to count the calories for a single 1½-ounce shot and then pour out very much more. And it is very dreary to have to measure precisely every sip or glass of wine.

For this reason, the number of calories in a whole bottle is often the safest and easiest guide to accuracy—and the most restraining influence—for home consumption. If you drink vodka, for instance, first decide how much to allow yourself for the week. Then set that quantity aside in a separate bottle. Those are your alcoholic calories for the week, and when you've finished that's your lot—so an overindulgent Monday could lead to a dry Saturday and Sunday. This way there is just no chance of making a multiplicity of little calorie mistakes with each drink, which could add up to many extra calories in a week.

Where wine is concerned, however, since it is purchased in bottles of so many different sizes, and at restaurants served in carafes (from minicarafes up to quart size), the best way to keep a record of consumption is to allow 4 ounces per glass, an average serving. This would be about

90 calories per drink. For home consumption, a week's quota can be poured into a separate corked or capped bottle. If you think you can limit yourself to four glasses, this would fill a pint bottle (16 fluid ounces), totaling 360 calories per week. A quart (32 ounces) would give you 8 drinks per week, 720 calories.

But don't forget to add in whatever is consumed away from home, both spirits and wine, at parties and at bars. When you've used up your week's quota, and want to preserve the illusion of drinking along with the rest, you could ask for Perrier water with a wedge of lime, which is still very chic. If the host or the bartender does not have Perrier, make it club soda or seltzer with lime or lemon.

In the following chart, calories are given for 25-ounce (750-ml) bottles of spirits (hard liquor) as well as standard 1½-ounce drinks, the regulation bar measure. Get out your calculator to estimate how many drinks you can splurge on per week—4 drinks of spirits (hard liquor) would be 6 ounces, ¾ of a measuring cup—and put that amount in a separate container. If you are a beer drinker, put your own mark on the number of cans or bottles you will allow yourself. Don't cheat!

Calories

Hard Liquor (Spirits)

Whiskey (bourbon, rye or Scotch), gin,
      vodka, or rum (86 proof)
      per fifth (25 fluid ounces, 750 ml)   1,860
      per drink (1½-ounce shot measure)   110

Wines

White, red, or rosé table wine, 4-ounce serving	90
Dry (cocktail) sherry, 2 ounces	85
Cream sherry, 2 ounces	100

Aperitifs and Mixed Drinks

Dry (French) vermouth, 4 ounces	105
Sweet (Italian) vermouth, 4 ounces	140
Dry martini (3½ ounces; 5 parts gin, 1 vermouth)	260
Whiskey sour, 3½ ounces	140
Daiquiri, 3½ ounces	140

Beers

Beer, 12-ounce can or bottle	160
Beer, 4.5 percent alcohol, 12 ounces	150
Light beer, 12 ounces	100

11

Fiber-Filler, the F-Plan's Built-in Slimming Aid

While following the F-Plan you will be able to choose from a wide variety of meals to suit your own taste in selecting daily menus. However, there is one dish that should be included every day. We call it Fiber-Filler. It's a kind of granola but much higher in fiber and lower in sugar. It provides exceptional filling power. We think you will be surprised at the remarkable effect this relatively modest-looking quantity of food will have in satisfying your appetite for really long periods.

Your daily portion of Fiber-Filler provides about 15 grams of dietary fiber, which is more than many people normally consume in an entire day. Most of this fiber is from cereal sources, which are particularly recommended for their health value by some leading medical researchers. But fiber from fruit and nut sources is included too.

To make your daily quantity of Fiber-Filler, mix together the following ingredients:

For one day

⅓ cup Bran Flakes (40 percent)
3 tablespoons bran meal
3 tablespoons Bran Buds or All-Bran
2 tablespoons sliced almonds
1 large pitted prune, chopped
2 dried apricot halves, chopped
1 tablespoon raisins

You will find it easier to multiply the ingredients, making several servings at one time. But if you do this, be sure to mix the ingredients well, for the bran tends to filter down to the bottom in its dry state. Divide into daily portions and store in separate plastic storage bags.

For eight days

2⅔ cups Bran Flakes
1½ cups bran meal
1½ cups Bran Buds or All-Bran
1   cup sliced almonds
8   large pitted chopped prunes
16 chopped dried apricot halves
½   cup raisins

Your daily quantity of Fiber-Filler looks relatively modest in a dry state, but once it is mixed with milk you will find that it provides two very satisfying servings, and tastes surprisingly good.

We recommend one serving (half the daily quantity) for breakfast; this will keep you comfortably free of hunger right through to lunch.

The remaining half of the Fiber-Filler plays an equally helpful role in aiding willpower. Save this to be eaten at any time during the day (in addition to your other meals) when you begin to feel hungry and vulnerable to eating temptations. Many people will decide to save it until suppertime. Evenings represent maximum temptation for most slimmers, although around four o'clock in the afternoon, when the children come home from school, can be the worst time for many mothers, who may be waiting until mid-evening to dine with their husbands. In these circumstances, this might be the best time to eat the remaining portion.

Yet another way in which you might choose to use the second half of your daily Fiber-Filler is to divide it into two portions and eat one of these half an hour before each of the two main meals of the day. This way it will act rather like an appetite suppressant pill—or, rather, in the way pills would act if they contained sufficient cellulose. Fiber-Filler does contain a generous quantity of cellulose, so you will be feeling considerably less hungry when you start each meal; you will be able to eat more slowly and be very satisfied with a diet-restricted quantity of food.

The daily Fiber-Filler, made in the quantities given above, provides a total of about 200 calories. The Fiber-Filler with skim milk and two pieces of fruit will average approximately 400 calories and 20 grams of fiber a day. These should be subtracted from your total allowance of 1,000 to 1,500 calories for the day. The 20 grams of fiber should be subtracted from your daily total of 35 to 50 grams.

Milk used with your Fiber-Filler should be taken from the daily ½ pint (1 cup) of skim milk. You will find that only a small quantity of milk is necessary and that half a cup is sufficient to accompany your full daily Fiber-Filler allowance (¼ cup with each portion). This will leave you another ½ cup of milk to add to tea and coffee, or, if you drink your tea and coffee straight, you can use the rest of the milk for other things—to blend with pot cheese (in place of the cream added to regular cottage cheese), to make cream sauce with mushrooms or other vegetables, to add to soup or mashed potatoes, or to drink as a beverage.

The Fiber-Filler is a most important part of the F-Plan program. However, if, on occasional days, you find yourself caught without the necessary ingredients, we list a few alternative breakfast ideas, and these mixtures can serve for between-meal snacks, too.

In addition to the breakfast menus we recommend, supermarkets and health food stores now offer a wide selection of whole-grain cereals and other high-fiber foods.

Ideally, however, you should breakfast on your half portion of Fiber-Filler every day for as long as you are following the program (or have it at mid-morning if you are one of those who hasn't much appetite early in the morning). Only when this is not possible should you turn to another of the high-fiber breakfasts.

If you want to finish your Fiber-Filler at one sitting, that's fine too.

Another use for the Fiber-Filler: You can carry a plastic bag containing enough for a coffee break or afternoon snack to still any hunger pangs you may feel away from home.

In this chapter you will find a chart that will serve as a ready reference for determining the dietary fiber and calorie content of a large number of foods suitable for your F-Plan program. The foods have been arranged alphabetically so you can locate them more easily.

A list gives the "top twenty" foods that are the best sources of dietary fiber, and another chart gives the comparative calorie and fiber content of various flours. (You can even have pancakes on the F-Plan! If you enjoy baking bread at home, make your own whole-grain breads or pizzas. Or you may have a pasta machine for making whole-wheat pasta.)

You will find many surprises in the long chart of calorie and fiber values. Some foods that you would expect to be high in fiber are not as good sources as certain other, seemingly softer, foods. And bran, that ingredient said to top all others in the *percentage* of fiber, is shown to provide 6 grams of dietary fiber in a realistic serving portion. How is this possible?

When you sprinkle bran over breakfast cereal you will understand. A quarter of an ounce, which measures 3 level tablespoonfuls, is about as much as you can palatably take in a single serving without feeling you are eating a bowl of sawdust.

Most people will eat bran only with breakfast cereal. Yes, there are enthusiasts who add it to hamburgers, stir it into squash, or beat it into a milkshake. But in this chart we are concerned with the way the average person will consume an average quantity of particular foods. We use bran only where it is palatable. This is the realistic attitude, because few of us go on eating anything we dislike for very long.

Why we eat what we do and how much we eat of each particular food is a fascinating subject. Because of their sheer bulk, many fiber-rich foods fill us up fast, a built-in quantity control. But we also tend to eat food in units provided by the manufacturer. Nature, too, does a neat packaging job, which influences the quantity we consume.

Where one unit is usually sufficient to satisfy the appetite and desire, we tend to keep to just one unit—one apple, one pear, one orange. Where Mother Nature has been meaner in her packaged quantity, with plums for instance, one unit does not have a built-in stop mechanism, so we often end up eating a good deal more than we would of a larger fruit. This has been taken into account in compiling the chart, too.

How we buy food also has an influence on how much we eat of it at any one meal. If we buy half a pound we tend to eat either half a pound or half that quantity.

The size of the dish or plate we use affects quantity as well, and this mainly accounts for the variation in quantities of breakfast cereals. Where a cereal is very light, like cornflakes, an ounce will comfortably fill the usual break-fast bowl. With Puffed Wheat an ounce would actually overflow in many bowls, so people tend to serve less than an ounce. Bran cereals and granola types are rather more weighty, so here people tend to pour out more than an ounce just so that it looks sufficient.

Price is another factor that influences quantity with some foods—mainly those we think of as protein foods. For example, most people will be quite content with a 2-ounce portion of shrimp, because they have become accustomed to eating a modest quantity of an expensive food, while with codfish, for instance, 6 ounces would be a more usual serving. This factor applies less with foods rich in dietary fiber, because these foods—happily—tend to be inexpensive. But it might influence the quantities of grapes or strawberries consumed, for instance.

The amount of work we have to do in consuming any particular food influences the quantity too—both chewing (where high-fiber foods score so well) and manual work. In an experiment with overweight people, scientists discovered that when the subjects were allowed to eat as much as they wanted, they ate considerably fewer peanuts in the shell than peanuts provided already shelled.

On the whole, the bulky form of foods rich in dietary fiber has a wonderful restraining effect on the quantity consumed—one of the great advantages of the F-Plan. But use self-control in relation to nuts (it's a good idea to buy them in shells), and take care with dried fruit—we have observed that some dieters make frequent sorties into the pantry to nibble a handful of dried fruit. This way rather a lot of calories can be consumed; the chart gives the number of calories for each piece of fruit or a specified number of pieces or cup measure.

Dried fruit has been processed to some degree, of

course. It is interesting to note how often foods become fattening only when man has had a hand in processing them in some way. The foods that are consumed very much in the way they were grown—many of the fiber-rich foods—are rarely fattening. It would appear that God did not intend us to be fat.

The Top Twenty in Fiber Foods

This list can serve you as a general guide. For more specific calorie and fiber content of particular foods, to estimate your daily and weekly quotas, refer to the long alphabetical chart that follows.

1. Dried beans, peas, and other legumes. This includes baked beans, kidney beans, split peas, dried limas, garbanzos, pinto beans, and black beans.

2. Bran cereals. Topping this list are Bran Buds and All-Bran, but 100% Bran, Raisin Bran, Most, and Cracklin' Bran are also excellent sources.

3. Fresh or frozen lima beans, both Fordhook and baby limas.

4. Fresh or frozen green peas.

5. Dried fruit, topped by figs, apricots, and dates.

6. Raspberries, blackberries, and strawberries.

7. Sweet corn, whether on the cob or cut off in kernels.

8. Whole-wheat and other whole-grain cereal products. Rye, oats, buckwheat, and stone-ground cornmeal are all high in fiber. Bread, pastas, pizzas, pancakes, and muffins made with whole-grain flours are an important part of the F-Plan.

9. Broccoli—very high in fiber!

10. Baked potato with the skin. (The skin when crisp is the best part for fiber.) Mashed and boiled potatoes are good, too—but not French fries, which contain too high a percentage of fat.

11. Green snap beans, pole beans, and broad beans. (These are packaged frozen as "Italian beans," though in Europe they are known as haricot or French beans.)

12. Plums, pears, and apples—because the skin is edible, and because all are high in pectin.

13. Raisins and prunes. Not as high on the list as other dried fruits (see #5) but very valuable.

14. Greens, including spinach, beet greens, kale, collards, Swiss chard, and turnip greens.

15. Nuts, especially almonds, Brazil nuts, peanuts, and walnuts. (But consume these sparingly, because of their high fat content.)

16. Cherries.

17. Bananas.

18. Carrots.

19. Coconut (dried or fresh—but both are high in fat content).

20. Brussels sprouts.

12

The Where-to-Find-Your-Fiber Chart

FOOD	Portion	Calories	Grams Dietary Fiber
All-Bran cereal	3 tablespoons	35	5
	½ cup	90	10.4
	(1½ ounces)		
Almonds, slivered	1 tablespoon	14	0.6
sliced	¼ cup	56	2.4
Apple			
raw	1 small	55–60 *	3
raw	1 medium	70	4
raw	1 large	80–100 *	4.5–5
baked	1 large	100	5
Applesauce	⅔ cup	182	3.6
Apricots			
raw	1 whole	17	0.8
dried	2 halves	36	1.7
canned in syrup	3 halves	86	2.5

* Important as dietary fiber is, laboratory technicians have not yet been able to ascertain the exact total content in many foods, especially vegetables and fruits, because of its complexity. Consequently, estimates vary from one source to another. Where differing estimates have been found, an approximation is given in the chart, as indicated by an asterisk. The same symbol following calorie content means the number of calories has been estimated, varying according to other added ingredients, especially fats and sugars, and to the size of the "average" fruit or vegetable unit.

FOOD	Portion	Calories	Grams Dietary Fiber
Artichokes			
cooked	1 large	30–44 *	4.5
canned hearts	4 or 5 small	24	4.5
Asparagus			
cooked, small spears	½ cup	17	1.7
Avocado			
diced	¼ cup	97	1.7
sliced	2 slices	50	0.9
whole	½ average	170	2.8
Bacon-flavored chips (imitation)	1 tablespoon	32	0.7 *
Baked beans,			
in tomato sauce (8-ounce can)	1 cup	180 *	16
with pork and molasses	1 cup	200–260 *	16
Baked potato, *see* Potatoes			
Banana	1 medium, 8″	96	3
Beans			
black, cooked	1 cup	190	19.4

FOOD	Portion	Calories	Grams Dietary Fiber
Beans			
broad beans (Italian, haricot)	¾ cup	30	3
Great Northern, navy	1 cup	160	16
kidney beans,			
canned or	½ cup	94	9.7
cooked	1 cup	188	19.4
lima, Fordhook, baby, butter beans	½ cup	118	3.7
lima, dried, canned or cooked	½ cup	150	5.8
pinto, dried,			
before cooking	½ cup	155	18.8
canned or cooked	1 cup	155	18.8
white dried,			
before cooking	½ cup	160	16
canned or cooked	½ cup	80	8
See also Green (snap) beans, Chickpeas, Peas, Lentils			
Bean sprouts, raw in salad	¼ cup	7	0.8

FOOD	Portion	Calories	Grams Dietary Fiber
Beet greens, cooked, *see* Greens			
Beets			
cooked, sliced	½ cup	33	2.5
whole	3 small	48	3.7 *
Blackberries			
raw, no sugar	½ cup	27	4.4
canned, juice pack	½ cup	54	5
jam, with seeds	1 tablespoon	60	0.7
Bran Buds cereal	3 tablespoons	35	5
	½ cup (1½ ounces)	90	10.4
Bran Chex cereal	⅔ cup	90	5
Bran Flakes cereal			
plain	1 cup	90	5
with raisins	1 cup	110	6
Bran meal	3 tablespoons	28	6
	1 tablespoon	9	2
Bran muffins, *see* Muffins			
Brazil nuts, shelled	2	48	2.5

FOOD	Portion	Calories	Grams Dietary Fiber
Bread			
Boston brown	2 slices	100	4 *
cracked wheat	2 slices	120	3.6
high-bran "health" bread	2 slices	120–160*	7 *
white	2 slices	160	1.9
dark rye (whole grain)	2 slices	108	5.8 *
pumpernickel	2 slices	116	4
seven-grain	2 slices	111–140	6.5
whole wheat	2 slices	120	6
whole-wheat raisin	2 slices	140	6.5
Bread crumbs			
whole wheat	1 tablespoon	22	2.5 *
Broccoli			
raw, salad or appetizer	½ cup (2 spears)	20	4
frozen	4 small spears	20	5
fresh, cooked	¾ cup	30	7
Brussels sprouts, cooked	¾ cup	36	3
Buckwheat groats (kasha)			
before cooking	½ cup	160	9.6 *
cooked	1 cup	160	9.6 *

FOOD	Portion	Calories	Grams Dietary Fiber
Bulgur, soaked (for salad) or cooked	1 cup	160	9.6 *
Cabbage			
white or red, raw, shredded	½ cup	8	1.5
white or red, cooked	⅔ cup	15	3
Cantaloupe	¼ medium	38	1 *
Carrots			
raw, slivered (4–5 sticks)	¼ cup	10	1.7
cooked	½ cup	20	3.4
Catsup, *see* Tomatoes			
Cauliflower			
raw	3 tiny buds	10	1.2
cooked	⅞ cup	16	2.3
Celery, Pascal			
raw, chopped	¼ cup	5	2
raw, chopped	2 tablespoons	3	1
cooked	½ cup	9	3
Cherries			
sweet, raw	10	38	1.2

FOOD	Portion	Calories	Grams Dietary Fiber
Cherries canned in light syrup	½ cup	55 *	1 *
Chestnuts, roasted	2 large	29	1.9
Chickpeas (garbanzos), canned or cooked	½ cup 1 cup	86 172	6 12
Coconut, dried, sweetened unsweetened	1 tablespoon 1 tablespoon	46 22	3.4 * 3.4 *
Corn (sweet) on cob kernels, cooked or canned cream-style, canned succotash (with limas)	1 medium ear ½ cup ½ cup ½ cup	64–70 * 64 64 66	5 5 5 7
Cornbread	1 square (2½″)	93	3.4
Cornflakes cereal	¾ cup	70	2.6
Crackers cream	2	50	0.4

FOOD	Portion	Calories	Grams Dietary Fiber
Crackers			
graham	2	53	1.4
Ry-Krisp	3	64	2.3
Triscuits	2	50	2
Wheat Thins	6	58	2.2
Cracklin' Bran cereal	½ cup	110	4
Cranberries			
raw	¼ cup	12	2
sauce	½ cup	245	4
cranberry-orange relish	1 tablespoon	56	0.5
Cucumber, raw, unpeeled	10 thin slices	12	0.7
Dates, pitted	2 (½ ounce)	39	1.2 *
Eggplant, baked with tomatoes	2 thick slices	42	4
Endive, raw, for salad	10 leaves	10	0.6
English muffins, *see* Muffins			
Figs			
dried	3	120	10.5

FOOD	Portion	Calories	Grams Dietary Fiber
Figs fresh	1	30	2
Fruit N' Fiber cereal	½ cup	90	3.5
Graham crackers, *see* Crackers			
Grapefruit	½ (average size)	30	0.8
Grapes white red or black	20 15–20	75 65	1 1
Green (snap) beans, fresh or frozen	½ cup	10	2.1
Green peas, *see* Peas			
Green peppers, *see* Peppers			
Greens, cooked collards, beet greens, dandelion, kale,	½ cup	20	4

FOOD	Portion	Calories	Grams Dietary Fiber
Greens, cooked Swiss chard, turnip greens			
Honeydew melon	3″ slice	42	1.5
Kasha, *see* Buckwheat groats			
Lasagne, *see* Macaroni			
Lentils			
brown, before cooking	⅓ cup	144	5.5
brown, cooked	⅔ cup	144	5.5
red, before cooking	½ cup	192	6.4
red (dahl), cooked	1 cup	192	6.4
Lettuce (Boston, leaf, iceberg), shredded	1 cup	5	0.8
Macaroni			
whole-wheat, cooked (¼ of 8-ounce package)	1 cup	200	5.7

FOOD	Portion	Calories	Grams Dietary Fiber
Macaroni			
regular, frozen with cheese, baked	10-ounce package	506	2.2
Most cereal	1 cup	200	8
Muffins			
English, whole wheat	1	125 *	3.7
homemade, bran with whole wheat	2	136	4.6
Mushrooms			
raw, "button"	5 small	4	1.4
sautéed or baked, with 2 teaspoons diet margarine	4 large	45	2
canned sliced, water pack (4 ounces)	¼ cup	10	2
Nabisco 100% Bran cereal (1½ ounces)	½ cup	105	4
Noodles			
whole-wheat egg, cooked	1 cup	200	5.7

FOOD	Portion	Calories	Grams Dietary Fiber
Noodles			
spinach whole wheat	1 cup	200	6
Oatmeal, cooked	¾ cup	212	7.7
Okra, fresh or frozen, cooked, sliced	½ cup	13	1.6
Olives			
green	6	42	1.2
black	6	96	1.2
Onion			
raw	1 tablespoon	4	0.2
cooked	½ cup	22	1.5
instant minced	1 tablespoon	6	0.3
green (spring, scallion), raw	¼ cup	11	0.8
Orange	1 large	70	2.4
	1 small	35	1.2
Parsley, chopped	2 tablespoons	4	0.6
	1 tablespoon	2	0.3
Parsnip, pared, cooked	1 large	76	2.8
	1 small	38	1.4

FOOD	Portion	Calories	Grams Dietary Fiber
Peach			
raw	1 medium	38	2.3
canned in light syrup	2 halves	70	1.4
Peanut butter	1 tablespoon	86	1.1
Peanut butter, homemade	1 tablespoon	70	1.5
Peanuts, dry-roasted	1 tablespoon	52	1.1
Pear	1 medium	88	4
Peas			
green, fresh or frozen	½ cup	60	9.1
black-eyed peas, frozen or canned	½ cup	74	8
split peas, dried, cooked	½ cup	63	6.7
	1 cup	126	13.4
See also Chickpeas			
Peas and carrots, frozen (10-ounce package)	½ package	40	6.2

FOOD	Portion	Calories	Grams Dietary Fiber
Peppers			
green sweet, raw	2 tablespoons	4	0.3
cooked	½ cup	13	1.2
red sweet (pimento)	2 tablespoons	9	1
red chili, fresh, chopped	1 tablespoon	7	1.2
dried, crushed	1 teaspoon	7	1.2
Pimento, *see* Peppers			
Pineapple			
fresh, cubed	½ cup	41	0.8
canned	½ cup	58–74 *	0.8
Plums	2 or 3 small	38–45 *	2
Popcorn (no oil or butter or margarine)	1 cup	20	1
Potatoes			
Idaho, baked	1 small (6 ounce)	120	4.2
	1 medium (7 ounce)	140	5
all-purpose white or russet	1 small (3 ounce)	60	2.2

FOOD	Portion	Calories	Grams Dietary Fiber
Potatoes			
boiled	1 medium (5 ounce)	100	3.5
mashed potato (with 1 tablespoon milk)	½ cup	85	3
sweet, baked or boiled	1 small (5 ounce)	146	4
See also Yams			
Prunes, pitted	3	122	1.9
Puffed wheat cereal	1 cup	43	3.3
Radishes	3	5	0.1
Raisin Bran cereal	1 cup	195	5
Raisins, seedless	1 tablespoon	29	1
Raspberries, red, fresh or frozen	½ cup	20	4.6
Raspberry jam	1 tablespoon	75	1
Rhubarb, cooked with sugar	½ cup	169 *	2.9

FOOD	Portion	Calories	Grams Dietary Fiber
Rice			
white, before cooking	½ cup	79	2
brown, before cooking	½ cup	83	5.5
instant	1 serving	79	0.7
Rutabaga (yellow turnip), cooked	½ cup	40	3.2
Sauerkraut, canned	⅔ cup	15	3.1
Scallion, *see* Onion			
Shredded wheat			
large biscuit (½ ounce)	1	74	2.2
spoon size (1 ounce)	1 cup	168	4.4
Spaghetti			
whole wheat, plain (¼ of 8-ounce package)	1 cup	200	5.6
with meat sauce	1 cup	396	5.6
with tomato sauce	1 cup	220	6
Spinach			
raw	1 cup	8	3.5
cooked	½ cup	26	7

FOOD	Portion	Calories	Grams Dietary Fiber
Split peas, *see* Peas			
Squash			
summer (yellow)	½ cup	8	2
winter, baked or mashed	½ cup	40–50	3.5
zucchini, raw or cooked	½ cup	7	3
Strawberries, without sugar	1 cup	45	3
Succotash, *see* Corn			
Sunflower kernels	1 tablespoon	65	0.5 *
Sweet pickle relish	1 tablespoon	60	0.5 *
Sweet potatoes, *see* Potatoes			
Swiss chard, *see* Greens			
Tomatoes			
raw	1 small	22	1.4
canned	½ cup	21	1
sauce (canned)	½ cup	20	0.5
catsup	1 tablespoon	18	0.2
Tortillas, 6″	2	140	4 *

FOOD	Portion	Calories	Grams Dietary Fiber
Turnip, white			
raw, slivered	¼ cup	8	1.2
cooked	½ cup	16	2.2
Walnuts, English, shelled, chopped	1 tablespoon	49	1.1
Watercress, raw	½ cup (20 sprigs)	4	1
Watermelon	1 thick slice	68	2.8
Wheatena cereal, cooked	⅔ cup	101	2.2
Wheaties cereal	1 cup	104	2
Wheat Thins, *see* Crackers			
Yams (orange-fleshed sweet potato), cooked or baked in skin	1 medium (6 ounce)	156	6.8
Zucchini, *see* Squash			

Flour Fiber and Calorie Chart

Those who regularly bake their own bread, pizzas, or muffins, or make pasta at home with a pasta machine, will find the following chart useful as a guide to the comparative fiber and calorie values of various flours. This chart can also serve you as a guide in selecting commercial breads. Look at the ingredient list on the label before purchasing to see which whole grains (if any) are included. The proportion is indicated by the order in which ingredients are listed; those in greatest proportion come first. Don't be fooled by the expression "wheat flour" if the word "whole" is not in front of it. This is another way of saying "white flour" and making it sound better than it is.

Flour	*Portion*	*Calories*	*Grams Fiber*
All-purpose white flour	1 tablespoon	29	0.1 *
	1 cup	467	1.6
Cornmeal, stone-ground	1 cup	404	16.5
Cornstarch	1 tablespoon	29	0.1
Masa harina (for tortillas)	1 cup	403	17
Rye flour (dark, whole grain)	1 cup	368	14.4

* See note on p. 61.

Flour	Portion	Calories	Grams Fiber
Rolled oats (whole grain)	⅓ cup	98	4
Whole-wheat flour (100%)	1 cup	384	14.4

Some Useful Calorie Charts for Foods with No Fiber

We have concentrated on calorie counts and fiber content in this book, since that's what the F-Plan is all about. But to complete your meals, and have all the food elements you need, you will be adding certain dairy products, meats, fish, and poultry to your meals—and none of these possesses any fiber at all. Neither do any of the fats and oils. The following charts should help you to select these no-fiber foods that are lowest in calories, and in portions allowable within your total calorie quota.

Meat and Poultry	Portion	Calories
Bologna	1 slice	130
Chicken		
livers	¼ pound	140
broth from mix	1 envelope to make 1 cup	12
light meat, chopped	2 tablespoons	46

Meat and Poultry	Portion	Calories
breast	½ (split)	104
leg (thigh and drumstick)	1	112
thigh	2	120
Chuck steak, broiled	¼ pound	352
Frankfurter, beef	1	125
	2	250
Ham, lean	2 thin slices	75
Hamburger	1 thin patty (2 ounces)	90
	normal patty (4 ounces)	180
Lamb, lean for stew	4 ounces	200
Pork chop, lean, no fat, thin sliced	1	170
Pork, lean	¼ pound	242
Rib roast of beef	1 slice (4 ounces)	320
Beef broth from mix	1 envelope to make 1 cup	8
Salami	1 slice	130

Meat and Poultry	Portion	Calories
Top round of beef	¼ pound	180
Roast turkey breast	1 slice	80

Seafood	Portion	Calories
Clams, minced, canned, drained	¼ cup	26
Codfish, broiled or poached	2 ounces 4 ounces	43 86
Crabmeat, plain, shelled	¼ cup ½ cup	42 84
Flounder fillet	¼ pound	86
Sardines, canned, well drained	4 2	160 80

Scallops
  bay
  large sea scallops
	
	2 ounces
	2 or 3
		
		80
		80

Shrimp
  fresh, boiled
  frozen, shelled
  canned, wet pack
	
	½ cup
	2 ounces
	½ cup
		
		91
		50*
		80

* See note on p. 61.

Seafood	Portion	Calories
Sole fillet	¼ pound	86
Tuna, packed in water	¼ cup	50

Eggs	Portion	Calories
Chicken egg		
boiled	1 medium	78–80
fried (1 tablespoon fat)	1 medium	108
scrambled	2 medium	160
Omelet, plain, in nonstick pan	2 eggs	160

Dairy Products	Portion	Calories
Butter	1 teaspoon	36
Cheese		
Cheddar, Swiss, or Parmesan, grated	1 tablespoon	28
cottage, low-fat	½ cup	48
	1 tablespoon	6
Edam	1 ounce (2 tablespoons)	87

Dairy Products	Portion	Calories
mozzarella	¾ ounce	53
ricotta	1½ ounces	58
Ice cream	1 scoop	174
Ice milk	1 scoop	137
Milk		
homogenized	1 cup	161
(Grade A)	2 tablespoons	20
buttermilk, from skim milk	1 cup	80
nonfat dry milk, reconstituted	1 cup	80
skim milk	1 cup	84
Sherbet, fruit	1 serving	100
Sour cream	1 tablespoon	30
Yogurt (low-fat)	1 tablespoon	8
	¼ cup	32*
	1 cup	128
Margarine		
regular	1 tablespoon	100
diet	1 teaspoon	15
	1 tablespoon	45

* See note on p. 61.

Dairy Products	Portion	Calories
Salad oil (including olive oil)	1 tablespoon	100
	1 teaspoon	33

13

Eating Out on the F-Plan

The F-Plan provides you with many easy-to-carry meals, such as sandwiches, so hopefully you will take your lunch to work with you while dieting.

However, you may wish to join friends or business acquaintances for lunch from time to time, and evening invitations to dine at restaurants or in friends' homes need not be passed up. It is unrealistic to imagine you will sit in a restaurant adding up calories and grams of fiber, and you certainly would not be so crass as to sit calculating the contents of food served you at a party.

So what to do? No one expects you to retire from society while you are shedding those excess pounds.

The answer is to use common sense. Before dining out, if you feel hungry, snack on your Fiber-Filler so you will not be tempted to indulge in no-nos. Then keep your calorie intake low by following these two simple guidelines:

1. Stick to low-fat foods.

2. Select very simple dishes.

The first is especially important, not only for reducing weight now but for controlling it in the future. The weight-conscious often choose the most fattening dishes on the menu, in the mistaken idea that they are being virtuous. No, no—they would not *dream* of having potatoes, bread, or a dessert. But they will select dishes swimming in butter or nibble shamelessly on cheese, believing that because it is high in protein it is slimming! Fats are the most fattening foods of all. Even low-calorie vegetables like asparagus and spinach no longer remain so if topped with hollandaise or added to a quiche rich with cream and cheese.

The old low-carbohydrate method of dieting contributed to making social eaters fat. The idea that only foods high in starch or sugar could be fattening has accounted for the consumption of many excess fat calories in restaurants and at parties, including high-protein foods like fat-streaked steaks, fried shrimp, fried chicken, and breaded pork chops.

Now people are just beginning to realize that fats are the dieter's number one enemy, while F-Plan dieters will learn that their best friend is fiber, as they pioneer in this new method of weight control.

The reason for guideline number two, "select very simple dishes," is that fats can lurk in disguise in all kinds of sauce-covered dishes and entrees. Avocado, for example, is very high in fat, and when you order it stuffed with shrimp salad made with mayonnaise, you are ordering one of the most fattening first courses on the menu, and could well be packing down more than 400 calories before you even start your main course.

All sauces, salad dressings, creamed soups, and concoctions made with cheese should be considered highly suspect. In your own home, you can stick to low-cal versions of sauces, use skim milk for creamed soups, even prepare desserts that have less than 100 calories per serving. But away from home, especially in restaurants, you can't be sure what has gone into those entrees that sound so glamorous, so play it safe and order only unadorned foods and avoid anything that has been fried.

At parties, the best plan is to take small helpings (if service is buffet style), and if you are served by the hostess, leave most of the more-fattening items on the plate.

The following will help you to make selections from a restaurant menu.

Starters

• Consommé is one of the few dependably low-calorie first courses. It's lovely and clear, so you can actually see that they have not sneaked in extra calories.

• You can't go wrong with half a grapefruit.

• A slice of melon, almost any kind, is within bounds, too.

• Fresh fruit cocktail (but be sure it's fresh, not canned).

• If you order shrimp or scallops, insist that there be no cocktail sauce, only a wedge of lemon.

• The salad brought to the table immediately, which is now the custom in most American restaurants, is a fine offering to satisfy your nibbling instinct—while others fill up on white bread or rolls with butter. Only instruct the waiter sternly to omit *all* dressing. You might enjoy a squeeze of fresh lemon juice instead.

Main Course

• Grilled whitefish is fine if you tell the waiter forcefully that it must not be swimming with butter. Send it back if it is!

• Broiled chicken is always safe—but not the skin; that's where the fat is.

• If you order hamburger, ask that it be cooked well-done so at least part of the fat will be drawn off before it comes to you. Most hamburgers are at least one-third fat. And no French fries! Don't even let the waiter bring them. You might be tempted.

• Seafood mixtures, as long as they are not fried, or in a

rich sauce. Avoid tartar sauce, drawn butter, other dips. Try fresh lemon juice instead.

• Omelets—you can't go too far wrong with these, unless they are made with cheese or topped with sour cream.

• For the vegetables, broccoli is always a good choice. A baked potato is permissible, of course (if you refrain from adding sour cream or butter). Almost any other vegetable will do as long as it is plain. Nothing fried!

Desserts

For many Americans, skipping dessert altogether is fairly easy, but if you feel you must have something to finish the meal with satisfaction, fruit is your best bet. Strawberries or raspberries, if in season, top the list—though no cream, remember! And no ice cream, which is very heavy in fat. Watermelon and cantaloupe are also good choices. Here are other possibilities:

• Fresh fruit sherbet, any flavor
• Baked apple (if you omit the cream)
• Frozen yogurt
• Jell-O

14

The Startling Truth About the American Diet

Probably no people in the world are more health-conscious than Americans. The unwary foreign visitor has to watch out or be trampled to death by the endless stream of joggers, male and female, sprinting down city streets as well as country roads in a quest for the body beautiful. Britons make resolutions every New Year's Eve to attend exercise classes, and maybe actually will get around to it someday—years from now. But American women not only sign up for courses at spas and exercise salons, many go to these places methodically several times a week, keeping charts of inches and pounds lost.

There is perpetual talk of nutrition, too, and not only in casual conversations; one is bombarded by it over TV and in the women's magazines. Everyone is warned to beware of cholesterol, chemical additives, polyunsaturated fats, and hidden sugars. These have become household words. From this one might expect the U.S. to have the healthiest population in the world.

But the visitor is also struck by the great number of overweight people to be seen wherever one looks, people who are grossly overweight, and many obviously still quite young. Statistics reveal that with all the modern drugs and vaccines available for the fight against disease, and regulation of water supplies and sewage, the prevalence of what medical science calls degenerative diseases is quite shocking. These are modern-day afflictions, caused by lifestyle, not spread by germs and viruses.

The middle-aged are afflicted by a great plague of illnesses related to environment, lifestyle, or diet, or a combination of the three. Men in their forties and fifties, in apparent good health, drop dead from heart attacks. Everyone seems to know at least one friend or relative who has fallen victim to cancer. Millions of older people suffer from diverticulosis. Even quite young people suffer from diabetes, arthritis, and obesity. Young athletes collapse from fatal attacks of coronary disease.

The fact that these illnesses and health problems are virtually nonexistent in Third World countries where people live on what grows naturally is reason enough to believe there must be a correlation between degenerative diseases and eating habits. But further, repeated surveys and studies have shown that when people from such countries and societies move to Western nations, living and eating Western style, gradually they become equally prone to the "big C's"—cancer and coronary disease—and all those other predominantly Western diseases. It looks as if it must be something we are eating—or not eating!

15

Thou Shalt

Not doing things is, in general, considerably more difficult than actually doing things. And much more dreary. We are wisely told not to smoke, not to drink much alcohol, not to eat all that sugar or salt or fat. All good advice, but all a matter of "thou shalt not."

Until recently, the only medically based "thou shalt" advice was on the subject of exercise. Thou certainly shouldst do that. The benefits in weight control are obvious, the benefits in physical health undoubted, and the benefits even in mental health becoming increasingly apparent. Physical exercise is becoming known as a valuable tool in treating depression, and if you find that hard to believe just try forcing yourself into a vigorous half hour's sport, jogging, or even just a brisk walk next time you feel low, and note the lift in your mood afterward.

But, exercise apart, the medical profession has been mainly concerned with telling us not to do things, rather than to do things, and banning things rather than advocating them.

Many foods we have been happily consuming for years and thought were good for us are now classed as "subversive." For example, dairy foods, eggs, and bacon are frowned on because of their fat or cholesterol content. And after people had been sternly warned to eat less sugar, science tried to help out by introducing several sugar substitutes—only to have each, one by one, denounced by the Food and Drug Administration as possibly cancer-causing, based on massive doses given to animals. (The title of one book summed up the prevailing situation: *Eating May Be Dangerous to Your Health.*) Such caution obviously arises from the need to minimize the risk of long-term adverse effects on health.

Nutrition specialists are always equally ultracautious about recommending a particular food or food element until after a massive amount of scientific researching, testing, and debating has gone on, often waiting for years until they give official sanction to a particular nutrition theory.

So when a large number of physicians who are regarded as top authorities in the nutrition field became convinced of the positive benefits of dietary fiber, you can be sure the evidence must have been overwhelming.

Today the medical establishment, in both Britain and America, is overwhelmingly in agreement regarding the benefits of increasing our present intake of dietary fiber. This change in attitude has come about after a long period when fiber was regarded as of no use because no nutritive benefit could be singled out. Nutritionists proclaimed the benefits of vitamins, minerals, and proteins necessary for growth and repair of body tissue. But dietary fiber had no food value. It was simply the packaging that enclosed the other goodies, and who becomes excited about packaging once it has performed its function?

When it became known that people in many undeveloped countries remained free of many major killer diseases of Western civilization, it was obvious that medical research into these illnesses should start by delving into the question of what these people were doing, or not doing. One of the things they were doing, it transpired, involved one of man's most private functions—emptying the bowels. Medical friends have told us that one very eminent medical researcher grows so enthusiastic when he shows color slides of stools excreted by rural Africans that comments like "Look—aren't they beautiful!" fly from his lips during his lecture. Beauty is in the eye of the beholder, of course, and what he is seeing in his mind's eye, after years of study into worldwide distribution of disease in relation to diet, is the stool of someone unlikely to die from cancer of the bowel.

Third World communities that remain free of our degenerative diseases have been found to live on diets that contain a much higher percentage of carbohydrate than ours—carbohydrate obtained from cereals that have not been stripped of their dietary fiber, fiber-rich vegetables (potatoes and other root vegetables), legumes, and fruits. The rural African or Asian, living on a diet like this, moves his bowels in a way that can only fill the constipated Western world with envy. Effortlessly, and daily, he evacuates nearly one pound of soft stool—the kind of stool that overwhelms our medical expert with its beauty. In striking contrast the Westerner passes only a quarter of that weight in much firmer, harder stool daily—and often not daily—and often only with difficulty.

The transit time—the time it takes for the food we put into our mouths to pass along the whole of the intestinal tract until the residue is excreted as stool—has also been found to differ enormously between us and them. In rural Third World communities the average transit time is one and a half days; in Western countries it is about three days in young healthy adults; among the elderly it can even be as long as two weeks.

But does this matter? Only a few years ago, in their efforts to quell the excessive and unhealthy use of laxatives, many doctors were insisting that it did not matter. "Go when the good Lord moves you" was the general attitude. "Some people move their bowels every day, others only once a week. Just do what comes naturally."

It is strange how attitudes have come full circle. People

used to have an instinctive feeling that all that waste matter hanging around inside them could not be doing them
any good—hence the popularity, at one time, of some
strange practices like colonic irrigation, and the excessive
use of laxatives, which was, and still is, condemned on
medical grounds. Then, because of these questionable and
unnatural methods, doctors began to insist that "regu-
larity" did not really matter.

Now modern research clearly indicates that a good
speedy transit time and daily effortless evacuation of soft
stool is indeed a vital protective factor in maintaining our
health.

Dietary fiber is what makes the waste matter from the
food we eat pass through us and out of us at the desirable,
speedy, natural rate. This is one of the main reasons why it
is now considered to be such an important protective factor in saving us from diseases of the bowel, like cancer.

Before you go on to discard the "packaging" with
Christmas-morning abandon (that is, eat those refined
starches), read in the next chapter about the links that are
emerging between dietary fiber—or the lack of it—and so
many of our Western degenerative diseases and com-
plaints.

16

Major Illnesses Linked with Lack of Fiber

Most people are now aware of the apparent link between a high level of cholesterol in the blood and the danger of heart attacks. This does not necessarily mean that cholesterol is the cause, certainly not the sole cause, of heart attacks. But clearly for those in stressful occupations or situations, it is wise not to include too many cholesterol-raising foods like animal fats in the diet.

The carbohydrate foods that are prime sources of fiber contain no saturated fats (of animal origin)—unless, of course, butter or meat fats are added in cooking or processing. So the F-Plan with its high-fiber foods is also a low-fat, low-cholesterol diet, ideal for those who have sensibly taken to heart the well-established benefits of reducing fat intake.

Dietary Fiber and Cancer of the Colon

There is a vast variation in the incidence of cancer of the colon in different countries throughout the world. In America and Britain it and cancer of the lung are the most common forms of cancer. There is little doubt, in the view of even the most conservative members of the medical establishment, that the cause of large-bowel cancer is environmental and that the factors involved are related to economic development. The greater the degree of economic development, the greater the incidence of cancer of the colon.

No other form of cancer has been found to be more closely related to the Western way of life—and the Western way of eating. Research is showing that diets that appear perfectly all right in other respects may lead to processes occurring within the gut that could increase the production activity or the concentration of cancer-inducing substances—carcinogens.

There are various ways in which fiber-depleted foods are now thought to be linked with cancer of the large bowel. First, the small stools of Western man may have a higher concentration of these cancer-inducing substances than the large diluted stools of the fiber eater. The slow transit rate of fiber-depleted diets is also thought to encourage the formation of these potentially dangerous substances within the body—and to leave them in contact with the gut for too long.

In short, the basic instinct that seemed to tell many people that they needed a "good cleanout," and that nasty things could happen while waste matter lingered around in the body, seems to have been largely correct. It was only the unnatural methods they used to combat the problem that were wrong.

Bowel cancer is invariably rare in communities passing large stools, and stool volume is always small in communities with a high frequency of bowel cancer. It is dietary fiber, of course, that affects this stool volume. For example, among rural Finns, who consume a relatively high-fiber diet, cancer of the colon is rare. They have been found to eat about twice as much dietary fiber as New Yorkers, among whom this form of cancer is rife.

Perhaps the most compelling evidence of all comes from studies of people who have moved from one country to another—Japanese who have emigrated to California, for instance—and adopted Western diets. Large bowel cancer is uncommon among Japanese eating their traditional diet, but it was found that, within a generation, Japanese eating the American way had developed a risk of large bowel cancer equal to that of Americans. This strongly endorses the "it-must-be-something-we-eat" theory (although genetic susceptibility to certain diseases may play a role, too).

The strong dietary links emerge from studies of communities with high and low incidence of this form of cancer. Those at high risk are eating a lot of fat and very little dietary fiber. Those at low risk are doing just the reverse. All the evidence available clearly suggests that excessive fat in the diet increases the risk of developing large bowel cancer and that fiber provides protection against it. The British Royal College of Physicians has gone on record as stating that "there are reasonable grounds for the statement that, in genetically susceptible persons, large bowel cancer could be favored by a fibre-depleted diet." (Though they add, of course, that other explanations for the prevalence of this cancer in Westernized countries are possible.)

This statement from such a conservative and distinguished authority certainly puts the idea that dietary fiber is beneficial well beyond the "crank threshold." For all sensible people it would clearly suggest that more thought should be given to the fiber content not only of their own diets, but of those of their children.

Dietary Fiber and Coronary Heart Disease

Coronary heart disease is essentially a modern Western disease and was rare, even in Western countries, until after the First World War. Today it is the commonest cause of death in the West. It remains almost unknown among rural Africans and is uncommon in most rural communities in Asia. The evidence suggests that a variety of factors in our modern Western environment—cigarette smoking, diet, sedentary living, stress—may be involved. In our diets, emphasis has for many years been laid on the intake of saturated fat as the major danger factor, but this is certainly not the whole explanation.

When a project researching the cause of this disease carefully examined a group of men in London, recording their way of life and following their subsequent history for twenty years or until they died, the strongest risk factor for coronary heart disease was found to be smoking and the strongest protective factor the intake of cereal fiber.

The dietary fiber connection is not in any way as clear and direct as it is in the evidence concerning cancer of the colon. But what evidence has emerged about dietary fiber certainly puts it among the "good guys" helping to protect us from heart disease, as opposed to the "bad guys" like animal fat and smoking.

The good guys so far seem to consist of a team of two.

Bad guys (factors that are thought possibly to increase risk of coronary heart disease): being overweight; smoking; suffering from stress; eating too much animal fat; eating too much cholesterol-containing food (like eggs); eating too much salt; eating too much refined sugar; sedentary living.

Good guys (factors that are thought to help prevent coronary disease): taking sufficient prolonged exercise; consuming sufficient dietary fiber.

One of the reasons for the beneficial effect of dietary fiber is that it reduces the absorption of cholesterol—but there are other ways, too, in which it would appear to perform useful functions in keeping the heart healthy.

The evidence in favor of dietary fiber as a preventive measure in heart disease is not strong enough to be conclusive at this stage, but is certainly strong enough to be thought-provoking.

Diverticular Disease of the Colon

This is another of those modern Western diseases that

seems to have mushroomed up from nowhere over the past fifty years. But only over here—not over there. It is almost unknown in Africa and Asia, while in the West, from being relatively rare as recently as the 1920s, it has now become the commonest disorder of the large intestine. It is said to be present, although usually without symptoms, in one in ten people over the age of forty, and in one in three over the age of sixty.

Constipation is now recognized as a major underlying cause of this disease—and fiber-depleted diets are recognized as the major cause of constipation.

It is the effort and pressure that the bowel-wall muscle has to exert in propelling onward the firm feces produced by a Western diet (rather than the soft and voluminous matter produced by fiber-rich diets) that has been found to be the cause of this illness.

In relation to diverticular disease the beneficial role of dietary fiber is very clear. Today a fiber-rich diet, often including bran, is not only advocated as a preventive measure, it is also widely used in the treatment of this disease. Since the advent of treatment with bran, fewer patients have required surgery for the complications of diverticular disease.

Dietary Fiber and Diabetes

Having read earlier about the rebound hunger factor involved in diets consisting of large quantities of refined carbohydrate foods, you will already have gained some clue to the role that dietary fiber can play in the prevention and control of adult-onset diabetes, particularly common among overweight people.

In Western populations a fairly large proportion of middle-aged people develop difficulty in utilizing carbohydrates in their diets. This difficulty is caused by a fault in the insulin production of the body. Insulin, as we have already explained, is necessary to control excess blood sugar. If blood sugar level rises too high, then sugar also appears in the urine and the person may be regarded as a diabetic.

As well as diabetics, there is a borderline group of people who are better classified as having "impaired glucose tolerance." Though only a small proportion go on to develop diabetes, these subjects have an increased risk of death from cardiovascular disease.

As we explained earlier, insulin response to the carbohydrate foods we eat varies with the speed of absorption of the carbohydrate. Any safe dietary food that delays the absorption of carbohydrates may be regarded as beneficial—and here, once again, is where dietary fiber appears in a valuable preventive and protective role. Carbohydrate foods rich in fiber are absorbed more slowly than those from which the fiber has been stripped.

It looks as if the adult-onset type of diabetes so common among overweight people is most likely to appear among those who eat refined low-fiber foods. Again, it has been found to be uncommon among those living on traditional unprocessed foods. In the United States, it has been found that a diet very rich in unrefined high-fiber starch plus pectin supplements has caused remission of the disease in 85 percent of the adult-onset diabetic patients on whom it has been tested.

This change of diet should not, of course, be attempted by diabetics except under medical supervision. However, more doctors are now recommending unrefined high-fiber foods in diabetic diets, and some experts believe that those who stick to high-fiber diets do not become diabetic. So fiber certainly seems to point the way to a healthier future.

17

Little Things That Mean a Lot

It is not the purpose of this book to provide a complete medical directory of all the illnesses that are attributed, at least in some measure, to lack of natural fiber in the Western diet. We simply want to emphasize that the medical indications for the need of more of this substance in our diets are strong and impressive. This is not just a passing fad.

If you have not been impressed by the very positive connection between a lack of dietary fiber and the incidence of cancer of the colon, and the possible connections between lack of fiber and heart disease, you are unlikely to rush off for a loaf of whole-wheat bread in order to prevent appendicitis or gallstones, just two of the other ailments associated with our fiber-depleted modern diets.

However, little things that affect our vanity often influence us more strongly than major things that could affect our health.

A very effective antismoking series on British TV drew attention to the fact that smoking gives you bad breath—and did not even mention lung cancer. Well done! And now medical researchers should investigate the connection between smoking and the complexion. At least one American survey has suggested that smoking makes the skin wrinkle sooner, though research seems to have stopped there. What a shame it has not occurred to the medical profession that the fear of wrinkles would be a prime motivation in encouraging at least the female half of the population to give up the weed.

It has occurred to us that mentioning some of the unglamorous little things that could happen to you if you don't eat the proper amount of dietary fiber might be the most effective way to encourage the practice.

For Starters—Varicose Veins

We all know what varicose veins look like. Those who haven't got them certainly don't want them, and those who have them already certainly don't want them to get worse.

The initial cause of varicose veins is not fully understood, but there are some eminent medical researchers, like Dr. Denis Burkitt, who believe that, in susceptible people, increased abdominal pressure caused by straining to pass small, firm, Western-style stools is a major factor leading to ugly varicose veins. Hurry off for the bran!

For Male Readers—Females, Too—Hemorrhoids

There is simply no sex appeal in a hemorrhoid. Surprisingly little sympathy, too, considering the discomfort hemorrhoids can cause. Wary sufferers have learned to suffer silently lest they raise stifled giggles rather than sympathy.

Considering the nature of the ailment, it will come as no surprise that one of the major causes is thought to be constipation and, again, the straining involved in evacuating a hard fecal mass. In recent years it has been found that a high proportion of patients suffering from piles require no further treatment once they have switched to a high-fiber diet and as a result pass soft stools that can be evacuated with minimal straining.

For the Youngsters—Bad Teeth

Most children are probably sick of hearing about bad teeth, but the guardians of their dental health will be interested to note that leading medical experts quite firmly advocate a fiber-rich diet that "encourages mastication," for the good of the teeth. Teeth were made to chew with. If they are not used in the way nature intended, they become more subject to dental disease and cavities. Chewing fiber-rich foods helps to keep the teeth cleaner and free of plaque in a variety of different ways.

After years of medical doubt, it is at last safe to say with conviction that an apple a day—along with the other fiber-rich foods you will eat on the F-Plan—does indeed help to keep the doctor away. And also the dentist.

18

The Ever-After Fiber Factor

Probably the most depressing words that have ever been pronounced about any reducing diet are those enthusiastic phrases from well-meaning medics along the lines of "This is a diet that you can follow for the rest of your life." Normal human beings will discard all thought of even starting any such diet—instantly! Who on earth wants to think of following a reducing diet forever?

Do not throw this book away. We are most positively not going to say anything like that. What we are going to say is simply that the parts of this diet that are easy and effortless and even enjoyable to you will become part of your normal eating in the future.

Quite probably you just didn't realize that peas, beans, and sweet corn are such valuable vegetables, and you will now eat them rather more frequently because you like them anyway.

Having tried Bran Flakes, you might well find that you like them just as much as ordinary "enriched" cereals, so high in sugar and low in fiber that they have been called sugar-coated vitamin pills. And if you find that sprinkling on just a little bran in no way detracts from your bowl of breakfast cereal, then you may be tempted to continue to do so.

Preferences between whole-wheat bread and white bread are largely a matter of habit. Having become accustomed to whole-wheat bread during your F-Plan program, you might well find that by the time you have got slim you have actually grown to prefer it.

Once you have shed your surplus weight you will be able to increase your food intake, and on a normal quota of calories it isn't at all difficult to increase your dietary fiber intake to 40 grams a day just by becoming aware of the fiber-rich foods—as you will during the following weeks. It is considered that something in the region of 40 grams daily should be quite sufficient to protect your health in all the ways that have been described, and to make it much easier for you to control your weight in the future.

If you are a parent, it is almost certain that your increased awareness of the value of dietary fiber will start to influence the foods you provide for the family—and thus their habits and preferences in the future.

The major Western degenerative diseases don't happen in an instant—like infectious diseases—but creep up on us slowly as a result of years and years of bad eating.

Although you will never know it, it could be that the slimming diet you are about to embark on will prevent your own children from suffering from cancer of the colon forty years from now. Quite a bonus, when you think of it.

19

The F-Plan Diet Rules

Here are the essential rules to follow in order to lose your surplus weight on the F-Plan diet:

1. Determine your total daily calorie intake at a minimum figure of 1,000 and a maximum of 1,500. Read Chapter 8 for guidance on your ideal dieting calorie total.

2. In choosing your daily menus, aim at consuming between 35 and 50 grams of dietary fiber. Figures are given with each meal, details in Chapter 9.

3. Have 1 cup of skim milk each day. This supplies 84 calories, which must be subtracted from your daily total.

4. Apart from milk, drink only those drinks that are negligible in calorie content. These are listed in Chapter 10. (If you find it difficult to diet without enjoying a moderate amount of alcohol, refer to Chapter 10 for advice and guidance on how this can be made possible.)

5. Have two whole fresh fruits each day, an apple or pear and an orange. No need to weigh these fruits; day-to-day variations will tend to balance out the calorie and fiber content. Subtract another 100 calories from your daily total for this fruit and add 5 grams to your fiber total. You can include additional fresh fruit in your daily allowance by using the chart on page 118.

6. Eat the daily quantity of Fiber-Filler—the ingredients and amounts are given on page 53. Divide this into two portions, each mixed with milk from the daily 1 cup; have one of these for breakfast and the other at any time later in the day. Since this accounts for around 200 calories, you

will automatically count this in your daily total, and add 15 grams to your daily fiber total. (Have one of the alternate breakfasts only if you don't have the ingredients for the Fiber-Filler on hand.)

7. Choose freely from the calorie- and fiber-counted meals on the following pages to make up the remainder of your daily calorie and fiber total.

8. Add low-calorie vegetables freely to any meals. You will find these listed on page 117.

This is all much more simple than it might seem from the above, necessarily precise, rules. It works out this way. Your daily milk, two pieces of fresh fruit, and portion of Fiber-Filler add up to a total of approximately 400 calories and 20 grams of fiber. Subtract these calories from your total for the day and make up the rest from meals that you can select from those on the following pages. Also, make up your additional 15 grams or more of dietary fiber from the meals—so that your total daily intake of dietary fiber is between 35 grams and 50 grams.

• If you are dieting on 1,000 calories a day, choose meals adding up to 600 calories a day.
• If you are dieting on 1,250 calories a day, choose meals adding up to 850 calories a day.
• If you are dieting on 1,500 calories a day, choose meals adding up to 1,100 calories a day.

When you eat and how often you eat is entirely up to you as long as you keep to the correct calorie total and aim for the right fiber total. Some people prefer to save a large proportion of their calories for a big evening meal, and others prefer to eat small meals more frequently. "Do your own thing" is excellent advice in dieting—because "your own thing" tends to be the easiest thing for you, and the diet method that is easy is the one you will succeed in keeping to.

The F-Plan meals on the following pages give you plenty of scope for both doing your own thing and eating your own thing, whether it is something as simple as baked beans or a sandwich, or something considerably more adventurous.

A Word About Your Weight Loss

From the day you start F-Plan dieting you will start losing surplus fat. But because you are eating fiber-rich food, it may be three or four days before the loss of that fat becomes apparent on the scales.

The reason is simply a minor fluctuation in the fluid content of your body. Remember, fiber-rich food holds extra water, so two or three extra pounds of liquid retained inside you can easily obscure that quantity of lost fat. Be patient. By the end of the first week's dieting the scales will start to reveal the true story of your excellent rate of weight loss, and from then on it will be downhill all the way to your ideal weight!

One little "adjustment" problem may occur as you switch to this healthier pattern of eating. Those who have become used to low-fiber food may suffer from a little flatulence for the first week or two. This problem should soon resolve itself as you adjust to the diet. If you do find this a particular problem during the early stages of F-Plan dieting, concentrate on the meals that do not have a high content of peas and beans until you have become accustomed to high-fiber eating.

There are others here and there who find pure bran too effective, even when it's consumed only in the twice-a-day Fiber-Filler. If this happens to you, simply omit the bran and double the quantity of Bran Buds or All-Bran—as long as the total amount of daily dietary fiber remains the same.

Important Health Note

If you are overweight but are otherwise in sound health, it would be unrealistic to ask you to get your doctor's permission to diet. However, if you suffer from any health complications it would be wise of you to tell your doctor that you are planning to follow a high-fiber, low-calorie diet, and ask his or her advice. Happily, dietary fiber in its natural state in food has not been shown to cause or exacerbate any human disease in the Western population, apart from high-grade obstruction within the alimentary tract or colonic disease. Its effect, as you have read earlier in the book, is to protect you from ill health rather than cause it.

II

THE F-PLAN MEALS

Introduction

The quantities for most of the meals on the following pages are given for a single serving. Our experience shows that dieters very often prefer to eat alone rather than at the family table—contrary to the exhortation "Make this for the family, too" beloved by many other diet experts.

As you read of the virtues of dietary fiber in the prevention of illness you will almost certainly want to introduce more fiber into the family diet. But for the dieter it is generally more helpful to have recipes in single servings, and if you like a particular dish so much you want to serve it to your family, you can easily multiply quantities with a simple pocket calculator.

When a recipe requires extra preparation time, or has a lengthy list of ingredients, and when it will freeze well, we give recipes for three or four servings. This is to save you time in the kitchen, a very hazard-filled area for dieters. The less time spent there, the better.

When you make up these multiportion recipes, immediately divide them into individual meal servings and either bag all of them, or put them up in small plastic containers with lids (all but the portion you intend having immediately for your lunch or dinner, of course). With the freezer well stocked with these individual servings, all you need do is take out two at a time for a day's quota, and you will have allowed yourself wonderful variety, with no need to grow bored with your diet. Be sure to label each with the name of the dish and the calorie and fiber count of each serving, so when you pick them out of the freezer you will know what you are getting.

When a recipe is given for two servings, you need not freeze the remainder; just keep it in a covered container in the refrigerator to have the next day or two days hence.

Similarly, if a recipe calls for half a can of chickpeas, measure out that much; put the rest away in the refrigerator in a covered container. Most canned products keep well up to a week if refrigerated. But do not leave food in the cans! Transfer to plastic or glass containers with covers.

Where it is most practical, we have used the entire contents of a can or packaged frozen product, even if this makes more than one serving. A 16-ounce can contains 2 cups, which in most cases supplies two normal servings. Many products are put up on shelves in 8-ounce cans for single servings, but it costs more to buy them this way. Frozen vegetables need to be at least partially defrosted before you can separate them into portions, so if you are using half now, put the remainder in a plastic sandwich bag immediately and refreeze. Or cook the remainder and store like any leftover vegetable in a covered container.

Most of the recipes and menu suggestions that follow have been grouped according to the fiber-rich food that forms the main ingredient of the meal. This should help you to use up half portions of processed foods.

We have rounded off calorie values of meals to make it easy for you to add together your 600 to 1,100 calories allowed for the day (in addition to your 400 from Fiber-Filler, fruit, and milk), and also the gram figures for fiber. Both are given for *individual servings.*

The meals are designed to cater to all tastes. They include some very simple meals as well as some more imaginative dishes.

Most of the soups are meals in themselves. If you want something more, add vegetables from the list on page 117.

Both the fruit and the yogurt desserts can be consumed with a clear conscience when you have calories to spare in your daily allowance. All provide fiber and other important nutrients, yet are low in calories. Remember, the pectin in fruit is a dieter's best friend.

Included at the end are daily menus to show how the recipes can be combined in high-fiber, low-calorie combinations to provide meals that will be satisfying, nutritionally balanced, and within your daily calorie quota.

About measurements. Standard cup and tablespoon measures have been used as follows:

3 teaspoons = 1 tablespoon
2 tablespoons = ⅛ cup
4 tablespoons = ¼ cup
8 tablespoons = ½ cup
16 tablespoons = 1 cup (8 fluid ounces)
2 cups = 1 pint (16 fluid ounces)
4 cups = 1 quart (32 fluid ounces)

The above refer only to *fluid ounces.* Dry weight measures differ from food to food. For example, an ounce of lettuce nearly fills a cup measure, while 3 ounces of cooked kidney beans measure only ¼ cup. For dry equivalents, 2 ounces = ⅛ pound, 4 ounces = ¼ pound, and 16 ounces = 1 pound. If a recipe calls for 2 ounces of ham, you would buy ¼ pound, then divide this in two, using half for each meal that calls for ham as an ingredient.

We have used convenience (processed) foods wherever possible to simplify food preparation. Instant minced onion can be used in most recipes that call for chopped onion, allowing 1 tablespoon to equal ¼ cup—if the food is to be cooked in liquid for at least 10 minutes (but not for salads or sandwich mixtures). Beef- and chicken-flavored mixes or concentrates can be used for making broth, or if you prefer, use canned beef consommé (diluted as specified on the can) or chicken broth. Imitation bacon chips (or bits) lend bacon flavor to bean dishes, salads, and sandwich fillings. These are a soybean byproduct, so they even add a bit of fiber (about 7/10 gram per tablespoon), yet contain no animal fat. (They are, however, quite salty, and therefore not recommended if you are on a low-sodium diet.) Several reduced-calorie salad dressings are now available and will help you to keep your calorie count within the quota. Herb Magic Italian Dressing contains only 4 calories per tablespoon. Some brands of imitation mayonnaise have only 40 calories per tablespoon, less than half as much as regular mayonnaise, and if you use only a teaspoon (as for sandwich fillings), that's a mere 13 added calories per sandwich.

A metric conversion table will be found on page 236.

Eating Extra Fruits and Vegetables on the F-Plan

Two pieces of fruit, an apple or pear plus an orange (to ensure Vitamin C), are included as a basic part of your F-Plan program. However, you can add extra fruit any day, as long as it's within your daily calorie allowance and this will, of course, add to your daily dietary fiber intake. For easy reference the calories and dietary fiber in popular fruits are listed below.

Many vegetables are very low in calories. Although some of them provide only meager quantities of dietary fiber there is no reason why any low-calorie vegetables should not be added freely to *any* F-Plan meal you choose. Each meal in this book ensures a generous dietary fiber intake. By adding extra low-calorie vegetables you will not be adding sufficient calories to slow your weight loss, so you can spare yourself the chore of counting the calories provided by these vegetables. But do remember to count the calories in any salad dressings you may add.

Below we list the low-calorie vegetables that can be added freely to meals or eaten between meals. Those that supply a significant quantity of dietary fiber are marked with an asterisk so that you can check with the calorie and fiber charts on pages 61–78 and add the grams of fiber provided into your daily total.

* Artichokes, steamed
  Asparagus (without butter)
  Bamboo shoots
  Bean sprouts, canned or raw
* Broccoli
* Brussels sprouts
* Cabbage
* Carrots
* Cauliflower
* Celery
  Cucumber
  Eggplant (not fried or cooked in fat)
  Endive
* Green (snap) beans

* Greens—collards, beet greens, dandelion, kale, Swiss chard, turnip greens
  Lettuce
* Mushrooms (when not fried or prepared with fat)
* Okra, fresh or frozen
  Onion (when not cooked in fat)
  Parsley
  Peppers
  Radishes
* Sauerkraut
* Spinach
* Squash
  Tomatoes (not fried)
* Turnips, boiled
  Watercress

Note: If you add really large quantities of these vegetables to your regular daily menus, subtract 50 calories from your daily calorie total.

Fruit Calorie and Fiber Chart

Fruit	Portion	Calories	Grams Dietary Fiber
Fresh Fruit			
Raspberries	½ cup	20	4.6
Blackberries	½ cup	27	4.4
Apple	1 medium	70	4
Pear	1 medium	88	4
Banana	1 medium	96	3
Peach	1 medium	38	2.3
Fig, fresh	1 small	30	2
Plums	2–3 small	38—45	2
Strawberries	½ cup	23	1.5
Orange	1 small	35	1.2
Cherries, sweet	10	38	1.2
Grapes, white	20	75	1
Dried Fruit			
Figs	2 medium	80	7
Raisins	2 tablespoons	58	2
Apricots	2 halves	36	1.7
Prunes	2	81	1.3
Dates	2	39	1.2

Pepping Up Your Meals

If some of these foods seem too bland for your taste, especially when you must omit butter, sauces, or salad dressings, remember you can always pep up flavor with herbs,

spices, or other calorie-free condiments. For example:
• add a sprinkling of dried basil or marjoram, or chopped fresh parsley to cooked vegetables.
• sprinkle caraway or dill over cooked carrots or beets.
• sprinkle curry powder, ground cumin, or ground fennel over chicken, fish, or eggs. Also add to low-calorie yogurt to serve as a salad dressing or sauce.
• add orange or lemon zest (the grated peel) to salad mixtures.
• lemon juice will enhance the flavor of almost any food.
• black pepper added to mashed potatoes will help make up for lack of butter.
• ground mustard, a pinch of cayenne or cumin will spice up bean dishes.
• nutmeg adds zest to spinach; anise or fennel will do a lot for the flavor of frozen peas.

The following can be used quite freely with any F-Plan meals: garlic, Worcestershire sauce, vinegar, soy sauce.

Breakfasts

F-Plan dieters should ideally breakfast on the half portion of their daily Fiber-Filler. These additional breakfasts are only for those who want an alternative if their Fiber-Filler mix has run out and some ingredients for making a new batch are missing.

PUFFED WHEAT MIX

Calories: 100   Fiber: 7.5 grams

½   cup Puffed Wheat
2   tablespoons bran
2   tablespoons raisins

BRAN FLAKES PLUS BRAN

Calories: 165   Fiber: 11 grams

1   cup 40% Bran Flakes
2   tablespoons raisins
2   tablespoons bran

KELLOGG'S CRACKLIN' BRAN WITH APRICOTS

Calories: 180   Fiber: 10.5 grams

½   cup Cracklin' Bran
2   tablespoons bran
3   dried apricot halves, chopped

KELLOGG'S MOST WITH ALMONDS

Calories: 190   Fiber: 11 grams

½   cup Most cereal
3   tablespoons almonds
2   tablespoons bran
1   tablespoon raisins

BRAN CHEX WITH SUNFLOWER KERNELS

Calories: 150   Fiber: 9 grams

½   cup Bran Chex
½   tablespoon sunflower seed kernels
1   tablespoon raisins
2   tablespoons bran

CORN BRAN WITH APRICOTS

Calories: 160   Fiber: 8 grams

½   cup Quaker Corn Bran cereal
1   tablespoon bran
2   dried apricot halves, chopped

1

Simple Hi-Fi Meals

Your meals on the F-Plan diet can be as simple or as unusual as you like. To show you how simple they can be, we start with meals that make use of foods that require no special recipes: meat, chicken, or seafood, which can be broiled, baked, or quickly cooked in small portions; familiar vegetables available in the frozen food section or in fresh produce; and salad ingredients that merely need be thrown together. A few are vegetarian meals, since many Americans, especially the younger generation, have turned to this way of eating. The vegetarian meals are the lowest of all in calories.

OMELET AU FINES HERBES WITH VEGETABLES

Calories: 350   Fiber: 8.5 grams

Omelet of 2 eggs beaten with 1 tablespoon chopped parsley
½   cup lima beans
4   or 5 raw carrot sticks
Salad of 2 sliced tomatoes and bean sprouts with sprinkling of oil and lemon juice, salt, and mixed herbs

MINUTE STEAK WITH PARSLEYED POTATO AND ZUCCHINI

Calories: 320   Fiber: 9 grams

¼   pound lean minute steak
1   medium (5-ounce) parsleyed potato
½   cup steamed sliced zucchini
⅓   cup applesauce with ¼ cup low-fat yogurt

TRICOLOR PORK CHOP DINNER

Calories: 440   Fiber: 18.5 grams

1   thin, lean pork chop (trimmed of all fat)
½   cup corn with minced parsley
½   cup peas
1   small sweet potato, baked or boiled

TUNA AND NOODLES

Calories: 315   Fiber: 14 grams

⅛   pound (¼ of 8-ounce package) whole-wheat egg
    noodles
¼   cup water-packed tuna
1   tablespoon chopped parsley
    Sprinkling of Parmesan cheese
½   cup cooked spinach
    Sliced tomato with 1 tablespoon low-fat cottage cheese

Cook noodles in boiling water until tender, drain, and add tuna, parsley, and cheese.

SHRIMP DINNER

Calories: 220   Fiber: 10 grams

2   ounces (⅓ of 6-ounce package) frozen shelled shrimp
    cooked with 1 small chopped tomato and 1 tablespoon
    chopped green pepper
1   small (6-ounce) baked Idaho potato
    Salad of 4 slices raw zucchini, 1 tablespoon grated raw
    carrot, and ¼ cup cooked green beans with 1 teaspoon
    reduced-calorie Italian dressing

ESCALLOPED TOMATO DINNER WITH SPINACH

Calories: 360   Fiber: 18 grams

    Escalloped Tomatoes with Cheese (see below)
½   cup cooked spinach
1   small baked potato
1   orange, sliced or diced, sprinkled with 1 teaspoon
    dried coconut

ESCALLOPED TOMATO WITH CHEESE

1½ cups canned tomatoes
1   slice whole-wheat bread
    Salt and pepper
1   teaspoon diet margarine
1   tablespoon grated Cheddar cheese

Put the canned tomatoes in a small baking dish; break up
the bread in small pieces and push down into the tomatoes. Sprinkle with salt and pepper. Dot with margarine.
Bake on same shelf as the potato for about 1 hour at
400°F. During last 10 minutes, sprinkle cheese over the
tomatoes.

TURKEY BREAST WITH BEETS AND CORN

Calories: 245   Fiber: 10 grams

1   thin slice of turkey breast (no fat or skin)
½   cup cooked sliced beets with vinegar and caraway
     seeds
     Corn on the cob
     Salad of ½ cup raw spinach with 1 teaspoon imitation
     bacon chips, 2 sliced raw mushrooms, and 1
     tablespoon reduced-calorie vinaigrette dressing

Thin slices of turkey breast that can be cooked like veal scallopini are now available in many markets, usually sold in the delicatessen department. Pound with the edge of a plate, just as for veal scallopini, then sauté over moderate heat in 1 teaspoon diet margarine.

CRAB LEG AND GREENS

Calories: 230   Fiber: 9.5 grams

1   frozen Alaskan crab leg, steamed
½   cup beet greens cooked with 1 teaspoon raisins,
     dressed with vinegar
½   cup mashed potatoes

When you buy a bunch of beets with fresh-looking leaves, save the leaves, trim stems, and cook like spinach in ½ cup water until quite limp, with 1 teaspoon raisins. Add a few dashes of vinegar to the cooked greens. For mashed potatoes, add 1 tablespoon skim milk and sprinkling of black pepper.

WINTERTIME SPECIAL

Calories: 215   Fiber: 10 grams

1   large parsnip, cut lengthwise
½   cup spinach
½   cup carrots with dill
1   teaspoon butter
     Cabbage slaw tossed with 1 tablespoon each sunflower
     kernels and yogurt plus salt to taste

Separately simmer each of the three vegetables very
briefly, or steam over hot water. Be extravagant—arrange
on a plate and dress them with butter.

BROCCOLI SUPREME

Calories: 200   Fiber: 15 grams

1   cup broccoli spears
1   small baked Idaho potato
2   broiled tomato halves with whole-wheat crumb
     topping

HAMBURGER AND VEGETABLES

Calories: 310   Fiber: 9.5 grams

¼   pound extra-lean hamburger, broiled
     Corn on the cob (with salt but no butter)
     Peas with mushrooms (½ of 10-ounce frozen package)

BROILED SOLE WITH BRUSSELS SPROUTS

Calories: 190   Fiber: 9 grams

¼ pound fillet of sole, broiled (one side only)
5 medium Brussels sprouts
½ cup chickpeas with parsley

BROILED CHICKEN AND LIMAS

Calories: 300   Fiber: 10.5 grams

1 broiled chicken leg, dusted with curry powder
½ cup frozen Fordhook limas with parsley
   Red cabbage and apple slaw

To make the cabbage slaw, combine ½ cup shredded red cabbage, ¼ cup sliced apple, 1 tablespoon chopped walnuts, and 1 tablespoon reduced-calorie Italian dressing.

SCALLOPS, SQUASH, AND BROCCOLI

Calories: 205   Fiber: 13.5 grams

3 large or 10 bay scallops, broiled with 1 small chopped tomato, sprinkled with herbs
½ cup thin-sliced yellow summer squash, sautéed with 1 teaspoon diet margarine
2 broccoli spears (½ cup)
   Salad of ¼ cup white beans with reduced-calorie Italian dressing

FRANKFURTER AND BAKED SQUASH DINNER

Calories: 250   Fiber: 9 grams

1   teaspoon diet margarine
    Black pepper
1   cup winter squash, cooked (or 10-ounce package
    frozen cooked squash)
1   frankfurter, split
½   cup green snap beans

Add margarine and a generous sprinkling of pepper to the
squash; put in small ovenproof dish. Top with the frankfurter. Bake in 350°F. oven for about 25 minutes. Simmer
or steam beans separately and serve with squash and
frankfurter.

ZUCCHINI VEGETABLE PLATE

Calories: 210   Fiber: 12 grams

½   cup sliced zucchini
½   cup sliced carrots
½   cup tiny cauliflower sprigs
1   tablespoon imitation mayonnaise
    Pinch of dried chervil or marjoram
2   bran muffins

Put the vegetables in a steamer, above boiling water, and
cook until barely tender, no more than 5 minutes. Serve
with imitation mayonnaise blended with the herb, accom-
panied by hot muffins.

TRICOLOR VEGETABLE PLATE

Calories: 210   Fiber: 12.5 grams

5 small Brussels sprouts
½ cup beets with reduced-calorie vinaigrette dressing
1 small sweet potato, baked in jacket
1 square cornbread

2

Sandwich Meals—for Home or Brown-Bagging

Whole-wheat bread and other whole-grain breads are important to the F-Plan. The calorie and fiber counts for sandwiches include the bread. You should have two slices per day or the equivalent in muffins or whole-wheat pita bread. Breads other than whole wheat that are acceptable include the mixed whole-grain breads, such as seven-grain loaves, sold at health food stores and some bakeries, dark European-type rye bread (but not regular commercial rye, which is made mostly with white flour), pumpernickel, breads enriched with bran such as Arnold's Branola, and, if you can find it, Boston brown bread. Authentic Boston brown bread is a steamed bread made of whole-wheat and rye flours and cornmeal. Whole-wheat raisin bread is also recommended; so are whole-wheat English muffins, whole-wheat pita bread, homemade bran muffins—and whole-wheat pizzas!

Besides sandwiches made with one of these breads, you will probably want to have toast or a muffin to accompany a salad or a vegetable meal. No butter is allowed, but for certain sandwiches, a single teaspoon (15 calories) of diet margarine is permitted, and you may sometimes spread a teaspoon of low-fat cottage cheese over bread or muffins, at a cost of just 6 calories. But *very important:* Do not spread with butter or margarine, not even diet margarine, unless the instructions say so, and don't use any creamy dressing but imitation mayonnaise in sandwich fillings—and be very stingy with that. Some brands of imitation mayonnaise have only 40 calories per tablespoon.

With a fiber-rich nutritious filling, a sandwich makes a satisfactory meal by itself, needing nothing more as a supplement than fruit or a raw vegetable snack. (See Eating Extra Fruits and Vegetables on the F-Plan, page 116.)

EGG SALAD SANDWICH ON PUMPERNICKEL

Calories: 215   Fiber: 5 grams

1 hard-cooked egg, chopped
1 tablespoon chopped celery
1 teaspoon reduced-calorie Italian dressing
1 teaspoon imitation mayonnaise
2 slices pumpernickel bread
2 tablespoons minced watercress

Chop egg quite fine; add celery, dressing, and imitation mayonnaise and blend well. If desired, add a bit of prepared mustard to taste. Spread half the egg mixture over 1 slice of bread, top with watercress, and add the other slice of bread.

BACON AND EGG SALAD SANDWICH

Calories: 255   Fiber: 7.5 grams

Use the same basic egg mixture as in the above sandwich, but blend in 1 tablespoon imitation bacon chips and 1 tablespoon minced parsley. Spread between slices of whole-wheat bread.

CHEESE AND CUCUMBER SANDWICH ON SEVEN-GRAIN BREAD

Calories: 335   Fiber: 7.5 grams

1   tablespoon reduced-calorie salad dressing
1   tablespoon skim milk
1   tablespoon sunflower kernels
3   tablespoons ricotta cheese
2   slices seven-grain bread
6   thin slices cucumber (not peeled)
1   teaspoon diet margarine

Add dressing, skim milk, and sunflower kernels to the cheese and beat until smooth. Spread over one side of bread. Lay cucumber slices over the cheese. Spread the other piece of bread with margarine. Put together. (If ricotta cheese is not available in your market, buy low-fat cottage cheese and add another 20 calories to the total.)

EGG, CARROT, AND PEANUT SANDWICH
(2 sandwiches)

Calories per sandwich: 210   Fiber per sandwich: 7.5 grams

1   hard-cooked egg
1   tablespoon reduced-calorie Italian dressing
¼   cup shredded carrots
1   tablespoon chopped peanuts
2   slices whole-wheat bread
2   tablespoons shredded lettuce

Separate yolk from white of the egg; beat egg yolk with dressing to form a paste. Add the finely chopped egg white, carrot, and peanuts; blend well. Spread half the mixture over a slice of whole-wheat bread; top with lettuce and the other bread slice. Save remaining filling.

TUNA SALAD SANDWICH (3 servings)

Calories per sandwich: 150
Fiber per sandwich: 7 grams

¼ cup (half a 7-ounce can) water-packed tuna, drained
1 tablespoon minced celery
2 tablespoons grated carrot
1 tablespoon finely chopped walnuts
1 tablespoon Bran Buds cereal
1 teaspoon imitation mayonnaise
1 teaspoon horseradish (optional)
2 slices whole-wheat bread

Combine all ingredients except bread; beat to blend and make as smooth as possible. Spread ⅓ of mixture between 2 slices whole-wheat bread. Refrigerate remainder of spread, covered; it will keep several days.

CHICKEN SALAD SANDWICH WITH APPLE AND ALMONDS (2 sandwiches)

Calories per sandwich: 190
Fiber per sandwich: 7.5 grams

¼ cup chopped cooked chicken
¼ cup minced apple (with peel)
1 tablespoon sliced almonds
1 teaspoon imitation mayonnaise
2 slices whole-grain bread
2 tablespoons shredded lettuce

Combine the chicken, apple, and almonds, add imitation mayonnaise, and blend well. Spread ½ of mixture over whole-grain bread. Add 2 tablespoons shredded lettuce and the other slice of bread. Keep remaining chicken mixture for next day.

PEANUT BUTTER, CHICKEN, AND CRANBERRY RELISH SANDWICH

Calories: 280   Fiber: 7.5 grams

2   slices whole-grain bread
1   tablespoon peanut butter
1   tablespoon cranberry-orange relish
1   slice white meat of chicken

Spread 1 slice of bread with peanut butter, the second slice with relish, with the chicken in between.

PEANUT BUTTER, CARROT, AND RAISIN SANDWICH

Calories: 240   Fiber: 8.5 grams

1   tablespoon peanut butter
1   tablespoon chopped raisins
1   tablespoon grated carrot
1   teaspoon diet margarine
2   slices whole-wheat bread

Combine peanut butter, raisins, and carrot; spread on 1 slice of bread. Spread margarine very thinly over the other slice. Fit together.

PEANUT BUTTER AND JAM SANDWICH

Calories: 290   Fiber: 8.5 grams

1½ tablespoons peanut butter
1   tablespoon raspberry or blackberry jam
2   slices whole-grain bread

The pure peanut butter sold in health food stores is preferable to commercial brands because it contains no honey or other sugar product. Or you may prefer to make your own, using a food processor. (See recipe below.) Raspberry and blackberry jam are both high in fiber, and so a much better choice than jelly, the kids' favorite, which has had all the fiber removed in processing, leaving nothing but sugar and fruit flavor.

HOMEMADE PEANUT BUTTER (12 servings)

Calories per tablespoon: 70
Fiber per tablespoon: 1.5 grams

¼   cup water
¼   teaspoon salt (if peanuts are unsalted)
1   tablespoon oil
1   cup dry-roasted peanuts

Put water, salt, and oil in blender or food processor (if using a food processor, oil may be omitted); with blender on, gradually add peanuts and purée. Makes ¾ cup; allow 1 tablespoonful per sandwich. Adding this amount to 2 slices of whole-wheat bread, you will have 195 calories and 7.5 grams of fiber per sandwich—if you add nothing else.

You can roast your own peanuts—buy raw peanuts in the shell, shell them, and spread over a pie pan in a 350°F. oven until evenly golden and crisp.

HOMEMADE PEANUT-CARROT BUTTER
(16 servings)

Calories per tablespoon: 60
Fiber per tablespoon: 1.2 grams

¼   cup water
¼   teaspoon salt (if peanuts are unsalted)
1   tablespoon oil
1   cup dry-roasted peanuts
⅓   cup coarsely chopped carrots

Follow the basic recipe, adding carrots along with the peanuts.

If using a food processor, for both recipes, all ingredients can be combined at once and oil omitted.

Hi-Fi Omelets and Scrambled Eggs

SUCCOTASH OMELET

Calories: 325   Fiber: 9.5 grams

½   10-ounce package frozen succotash
2   eggs, beaten
2   tablespoons skim milk
     Dash of Worcestershire sauce
¼   teaspoon salt
     Freshly ground black pepper
1   tablespoon imitation bacon chips
1   slice pumpernickel bread
     Watercress sprigs

Thaw succotash by putting in tightly covered saucepan over very low heat; break up with fork. Divide in half; store half in a covered dish in refrigerator. Combine eggs with milk, Worcestershire sauce, and half the salt. Pour the eggs into a nonstick omelet pan, cook until they begin to set, then add the succotash and sprinkle with remaining salt and pepper. Lift up omelet with spatula, to allow moist egg to run under. When it is almost firm throughout, but still somewhat moist, roll out of the pan onto a heated plate. Garnish with chips and watercress sprigs. Serve with bread.

MEXICAN SCRAMBLED EGGS WITH AVOCADO AND KIDNEY BEANS

Calories: 375 Fiber: 9.5 grams

2	eggs
1	tablespoon skim milk
¼	teaspoon salt
¼	cup diced avocado
¼	cup kidney beans, canned or cooked, well drained
½	teaspoon chili powder
1	slice whole-wheat bread
1	tablespoon low-fat cottage cheese

Beat eggs with milk; add ⅛ teaspoon salt. Pour into non-stick pan. When partially set, add avocado and beans and sprinkle with chili powder. Stir eggs to mix. Serve immediately on toasted bread spread with cottage cheese.

ARTICHOKE AND PIMENTO OMELET

Calories: 300 Fiber: 11 grams

6	canned artichoke hearts, drained and chopped
2	tablespoons chopped pimento
¼	teaspoon marjoram
1	tablespoon chopped parsley
1	tablespoon skim milk
2	eggs, beaten
⅛	teaspoon salt
1	square cornbread

Chop artichoke hearts coarsely; combine with pimento and herbs. Add skim milk to eggs with the salt; pour into nonstick omelet pan over moderate heat. When eggs have started to set, add the artichoke and pimento and lift up omelet with spatula to allow moist egg to run under. As bottom firms, turn over, and when firm but still soft, slip out onto warm plate. Serve with cornbread.

ITALIAN VEGETABLE OMELET

Calories: 440   Fiber: 17.5 grams

1 tablespoon diet margarine
2 tablespoons minced onion
2 tablespoons green pepper
¼ cup thinly sliced zucchini
¼ cup shredded carrot
½ cup canned or cooked kidney beans, well drained
¼ teaspoon Italian herb seasoning
2 eggs
   Salt and pepper
1 whole-wheat English muffin

Melt margarine in nonstick omelet pan, add onion, green pepper, and zucchini, and cook over moderate heat until soft but not browned. Add remaining vegetables, cook 2 minutes, and sprinkle with herbs. Beat eggs with 1 tablespoon water and ¼ teaspoon salt; pour over half the vegetables, lifting up egg with spatula as it firms. Add remaining egg; repeat. When firm but still moist throughout, invert onto plate, then slide back into pan, moist side down, and cook until lightly browned on the other side. Serve with toasted muffin.

SCRAMBLED EGGS, ALMONDS, AND MUSHROOMS

Calories: 330   Fiber: 8 grams

- ½ cup sliced mushrooms
- 2   tablespoons sliced almonds
- 1   tablespoon diet margarine
- ¼   teaspoon salt
     Dash of paprika
- 2   eggs, beaten
- 1   tablespoon skim milk
- 1   slice whole-wheat bread, toasted
- 1   tablespoon low-fat cottage cheese

Gently cook mushrooms and almonds in margarine in a nonstick omelet pan, turning as they brown. Sprinkle with salt and paprika. Beat the eggs with the milk and pour over the mushrooms half at a time, lifting up to allow moist egg to run under; cook until just set. Serve with toast spread with cottage cheese.

SPINACH OMELET WITH MUSHROOMS

Calories: 360   Fiber: 12.5 grams

- 2   medium eggs
- ½   cup thawed chopped spinach
- ¼   teaspoon salt
     Pinch of nutmeg
- 2   teaspoons diet margarine
- ¼   cup sliced raw mushrooms
- 2   bran muffins

Separate eggs. Defrost spinach by putting in heavy saucepan over very low heat, breaking up with fork; then carefully drain off all liquid. Measure out ½ cup spinach and refrigerate the rest in covered container for another recipe. Add salt and nutmeg. Beat egg yolks until somewhat thickened and add to spinach. Beat whites until stiff, then fold into spinach-yolk mixture. Melt margarine in nonstick omelet pan over moderate heat; add mushrooms and cook until lightly browned. Pour the egg mixture over the mushrooms and cook until bottom is set. Broil, 4 to 6 inches from heat, just until top is firm and delicately browned. Serve with bran muffins.

SPANISH POTATO OMELET

Calories: 385   Fiber: 8 grams

1   teaspoon olive oil
1   teaspoon diet margarine
½   cup finely diced raw potato
½   cup minced onion
2   eggs, beaten
1   slice whole-wheat bread, toasted

Heat oil and margarine together in nonstick omelet pan; add potato and onion and cook over moderate heat, turning occasionally, until soft but not browned. Add eggs, ⅓ at a time, to potatoes, turning up to allow moist egg to run under. When all egg has been added, invert on plate, then slide back, moist side down, to cook on other side. Serve with whole-wheat toast.

4

Potato and Other Hi-Fi Vegetable Combinations

Baked potatoes are an F-Plan favorite: easy to prepare, high in fiber, and everybody likes them. We allow for a smallish Idaho in the F-Plan meals. Since Idaho potatoes run fairly large, a "small Idaho" will run about 6 ounces. This is a potato about 3½ inches long. It provides 120 calories and 4.5 grams of fiber. For a 7-ounce Idaho, one that could be considered medium-sized, the calorie count goes up to 140 calories and 5 grams of fiber.

General-purpose potatoes, both the russet and the white-skinned, are rounder and more varied in size. A "small" potato of this variety may be no more than 4 ounces, only 80 calories, but only 3 grams of fiber. A medium potato would be 5 ounces (three to a pound), providing 3.5 grams fiber. These are best for boiling, mashing, for salad and omelets.

The usual way to bake a potato is to put it in the center of an oven set at 400°F. Allow 45 minutes to 1 hour to bake; you know it's done when it is pierced easily with a fork. To speed cooking time, you can put the whole unpeeled potato in a pan of water, bring the water to a boil, simmer 20 minutes, then remove, pat dry, and put in the oven for 10 to 15 minutes. Or, if you have a microwave oven, prick the potato all over and cook it at full power for 4 minutes, turning after 2 minutes.

Mashed potatoes can be prepared from instant potato mix, following label instructions for 1 serving. If the label gives no preparation instructions for less than 2 servings, simply divide these ingredients in half.

Potatoes can go into soup, salads, and stews for your F-Plan—but never fried. No French fries, no home fries—absolutely forbidden!

HAMBURGER AND PARSLEYED POTATO DINNER

Calories: 340   Fiber: 13.5 grams

1   medium (5-ounce) all-purpose potato
1   tablespoon chopped parsley
¼   pound extra-lean ground beef
½   cup frozen green peas (half a 10-ounce package)

Cook potato until fork-tender (about 20 minutes), drain, immediately add parsley. After potato has been cooking 15 minutes, broil the hamburger patty, and cook the frozen peas. If desired, season the peas with a pinch of anise or mint. (To make the potato more interesting, you may wish to top it with a tablespoon of yogurt, for an additional 8 calories.)

BROILED CHICKEN AND BAKED POTATO DINNER

Calories: 315   Fiber: 11 grams

1   small Idaho potato, baked
1   chicken leg, broiled
½   cup frozen or canned corn
4   carrot sticks
    Sauce for potato: 2 tablespoons yogurt mixed with chives

BAKED POTATO AND MEDITERRANEAN-STYLE FISH STEW

Calories: 240   Fiber: 6.5 grams

¼   pound fillet of cod or scrod
½   cup canned tomatoes, chopped
2   tablespoons chopped onion or ½
      teaspoon instant minced onion
½   teaspoon paprika
¼   teaspoon garlic salt
      Pinch of basil or oregano
      Freshly ground black pepper
2   tablespoons chopped green pepper
1   small Idaho potato

Put fish, tomatoes, onion, seasonings, and green pepper in small ovenproof baking dish with cover. Bake in 400°F. oven alongside the potato, for 45 minutes to 1 hour.

BAKED POTATO WITH HAM SALAD

Calories: 280   Fiber: 10 grams

1   small (6-ounce) Idaho potato
¼   cup chopped lean ham
½   cup shredded white or green cabbage
¼   cup grated carrot
1   small stalk celery, chopped
1   tablespoon minced parsley
1   tablespoon low-fat yogurt
1   tablespoon reduced-calorie Italian dressing

Bake the potato at 400°F. for 45 minutes to 1 hour. Mix remaining ingredients into a salad to serve with the potato.

HOT POTATO AND VEGETABLE SALAD

Calories: 240   Fiber: 11.5 grams

1   small red or white new potato
¼   cup frozen Fordhook limas
½   teaspoon salt
1   medium carrot, sliced
2   broccoli spears
1   teaspoon reduced-calorie Italian dressing
1   tablespoon imitation mayonnaise

Cut unpeeled potato in quarters to hasten cooking. Put in saucepan with limas, add 1 cup water and the salt, and cook until tender. Separately cook the carrot and the broccoli, both until barely tender, still a little crisp. Arrange the hot cooked vegetables on a plate. Beat together the dressing and imitation mayonnaise and spoon over the vegetables.

See also Swedish Potato Salad, page 179.

ASPARAGUS DINNER

Calories: 170   Fiber: 11.5 grams

6   trimmed asparagus spears
1   medium (5-ounce) potato, cooked in jacket
½   cup cooked carrots, seasoned with caraway seeds
¾   cup strawberries for dessert

Meals with Corn

CORN ON THE COB DINNER

Calories: 220   Fiber: 13.5 grams

1   small (4-ounce) russet potato
    Salt and pepper
1   small tomato, cut in half
    Italian herb seasoning
1   tablespoon fine dry whole-wheat bread crumbs
1   teaspoon diet margarine
1   medium ear of corn
4   thin carrot sticks
2   tiny raw cauliflower sprigs

Quarter potato, cook in salted boiling water until tender, about 20 minutes; drain, season with salt and black pepper. As potato cooks, broil tomato halves: sprinkle with salt, herb seasoning, and crumbs; dot with margarine. Cook corn in boiling water for 5 to 7 minutes; drain. Serve the three vegetables on the same plate; serve the raw carrot sticks and cauliflower separately as a salad.

CORN AND BEAN CHOWDER (2 servings)

Calories per serving: 220   Fiber per serving: 11.5 grams

1   cup (8-ounce can) cream-style corn
½   small potato, cooked, diced
1   tablespoon instant minced onion, reconstituted in 2
    tablespoons water, or chopped fresh onion to taste
½   cup kidney beans (canned or cooked)

1   teaspoon dried mustard
1½   cups skim milk
2   tablespoons bacon-flavored chips
     Salt and pepper to taste

Use leftover potato for this chowder; or, if you don't have any on hand, quarter a small potato, cook in salted water until tender, drain, use half of it (removing skin) in the chowder, and save the remainder for a mixed vegetable salad.

Combine corn, potato, onion, beans, and mustard. Divide mixture in half; put away one portion for tomorrow. Heat the rest in a saucepan, simmering 5 minutes at low heat. Add ¾ cup milk; continue to simmer but do not boil. Serve topped with 1 tablespoon bacon chips. (When reheating the remaining second serving, add another ¾ cup milk and top with 1 tablespoon bacon chips.)

CORN AND BEAN CHOWDER WITH CHICKEN

Calories: 275   Fiber: 11.5 grams

When heating the second serving of the chowder, add 2 tablespoons chopped cooked chicken (or turkey) along with the milk.

CORN AND TOMATO CASSEROLE

Calories: 320   Fiber: 14 grams

½   cup corn, canned or scraped from ear
2   tablespoons minced lean ham
1   small tomato, chopped
2   tablespoons chopped fresh onion
¼   cup frozen or cooked green peas
½   teaspoon dried basil
    Salt and pepper
¼   cup fine dry whole-grain bread crumbs
1   thin slice mozzarella or low-calorie cheese

Combine corn, ham, tomato, onion, and peas. Season with basil and salt and pepper. Heat in saucepan, simmer 4 minutes. Spread out over Pyrex pie pan. Spread crumbs over vegetables; lay slice of cheese over top. Broil, 4 inches from heat, until cheese is melted.

MEALS WITH OKRA AND EGGPLANT

OKRA AND PORK CHOP DINNER

Calories: 315   Fiber: 5 grams

¼   pound (about ½ cup) fresh okra pods, sliced
1   tablespoon diet margarine
    Salt
1   thin lean pork chop (4 ounces), all fat removed
1   small (4-ounce) potato
1   tablespoon minced parsley

Cook the okra in a nonstick pan with the margarine, stirring constantly to prevent browning, about 3 minutes. Sprinkle with a dash of salt. The chop can be pan-broiled: Lightly grease the bottom of small skillet just enough to prevent sticking, then cook meat until lightly browned on each side. Boil the potato in its jacket; when tender, drain, dice, and immediately add parsley.

SHRIMP GUMBO FOR ONE

Calories: 215   Fiber: 11.5 grams

¼ cup thinly sliced onion
1 small clove garlic, crushed
   Pinch of thyme
½ bay leaf, crushed
⅛ teaspoon crushed red pepper flakes
1 cup canned tomatoes, chopped
   Salt to taste
1 cup okra pods, sliced
2 ounces frozen shrimp (⅓ of 6-ounce package)
½ cup cooked brown rice or bulgur

Combine onion, garlic, herbs, red pepper, tomatoes, and salt. Simmer 30 minutes. Add okra and cook 10 minutes, uncovered, until sauce is thickened. Add shrimp and cook just until shrimp turn pink; do not let sauce come to boil. Serve with brown rice or bulgur.

GREEK-STYLE LAMB STEW WITH OKRA

Calories: 330   Fiber: 11 grams

1   tablespoon chopped onion
     Pinch of thyme
1   teaspoon olive oil
¼   teaspoon salt
1   cup canned tomatoes, puréed in blender
¼   pound boned lamb for stew
1   cup fresh or frozen whole okra pods
     Few drops lemon juice
½   cup cooked brown rice

Cook the onion and thyme in oil until soft but not browned. Sprinkle with salt. Add to tomatoes and lamb in saucepan. Simmer, covered, until lamb is tender, about 1 hour. (Cut up lamb into very small pieces to speed cooking.) Add okra and lemon juice in last 15 minutes. Serve with brown rice.

BAKED EGGPLANT CASSEROLE

Calories: 225   Fiber: 13 grams

1   cup diced peeled eggplant
1   tomato, diced
2   tablespoons minced green pepper
½   cup green snap beans, broken into pieces
½   teaspoon basil
¼   teaspoon oregano
     Salt
1   tablespoon diet margarine
1   small (6-ounce) Idaho potato

Combine eggplant, tomato, green pepper, beans, herbs, and salt in small casserole. Dot with margarine. Cover and put in 400°F. oven, alongside baking potato. Bake 45 minutes to 1 hour, until potato is fork-tender.

MEALS WITH SPINACH AND OTHER HI-FI GREENS

POACHED EGG OVER SPINACH ON TOAST

Calories: 160   Fiber: 8 grams

1½ cups raw spinach or ½ cup frozen chopped spinach
⅛   teaspoon salt
    Dash of nutmeg
    Dash of vinegar or lemon juice
1   slice whole-grain bread, toasted
1   large egg
    Salt and paprika

If using raw spinach, wash it thoroughly several times to get rid of all grit, then chop; cook it in just the water that clings to the leaves, until just wilted, about 2 minutes. Press out all water, pushing spinach against saucepan with spoon. If using frozen spinach, heat with 1 tablespoon water in small covered pan, stirring to break up, then thoroughly drain off all liquid. Season with salt and nutmeg. Add vinegar or lemon juice. Spread over toast. Poach the egg, place over spinach; sprinkle with salt and paprika.

BAKED SPINACH AND COTTAGE CHEESE

Calories: 200   Fiber: 8.5 grams

1½ cups raw spinach or ½ cup frozen chopped spinach
   Salt and nutmeg
½   cup low-fat cottage cheese
¼   cup fine dry whole-wheat bread crumbs
1   tablespoon grated Parmesan cheese

Prepare spinach as in previous recipe, seasoning with salt
and nutmeg. Spread over bottom of small (2-cup) casserole. Cover with cottage cheese, then the crumbs mixed
with Parmesan. Broil until crumbs are browned.

CREPES FLORENTINE

Calories: 400   Fiber: 9 grams

½   10-ounce package frozen chopped spinach
⅛   teaspoon salt
    Dash of nutmeg
1¼ cups skim milk
1   tablespoon whole-wheat flour
2   tablespoons shredded Swiss cheese
½   cup Aunt Jemima whole-wheat pancake mix
1   egg, beaten
¼   teaspoon diet margarine

Thaw the spinach; add salt and nutmeg. Measure out ½
cup milk; blend a little of it with flour until smooth; add
rest of ½ cup milk and the cheese. Heat, stirring with a
whisk, until sauce is thickened and smooth. Season to taste
with additional salt and pepper. Add half the sauce to the
spinach and keep it warm.

Beat the pancake mix with the remaining ¾ cup milk and the beaten egg. Grease a small (6- or 7-inch) skillet with just enough margarine to glaze the surface. (If you have a nonstick pan, this step may be omitted.) Pour out 1 tablespoon batter at a time, rolling the pan so it spreads out into a circle. When firm on one side, flip to cook on the other. Continue until batter is used. Put a tablespoon of spinach mixture in each crêpe, roll up, and place, over-lapped side down, in shallow casserole or Pyrex pie pan. Cover with remaining cheese sauce. Broil until sauce is lightly browned. (Crêpes can be frozen, to be reheated later in a microwave oven, or in a regular oven at moderate heat.)

KALE WITH BACON BITS

Calories for meal: 240   Fiber for meal: 9 grams

1   teaspoon sugar
1   tablespoon vinegar
¼   teaspoon salt
    Pinch of celery seed
¼   cup water
1   cup fresh kale or ½ package frozen kale
1   tablespoon imitation bacon chips
1   boiled or mashed potato
1   thin (2-ounce) hamburger

Add sugar, vinegar, salt, and celery seed to water; bring to a boil, add kale, and cook until kale is completely wilted, about 10 minutes. Drain thoroughly, pressing out all liquid, chop, and serve topped with bacon chips. To complete the meal, serve with boiled or ½ cup mashed potato and a pan-broiled burger. (Count for prepared kale alone is 70 calories, with 4.5 grams of fiber.)

COLLARD GREENS WITH RAISINS AND NUTS

Calories: 255   Fiber: 10 grams

1 cup fresh collard greens or ½ package frozen collard greens, thawed
½ cup water
  Salt
1 tablespoon raisins
1 tablespoon chopped peanuts
1 teaspoon vinegar
1 thin slice of ham
½ cup limas

Put collard greens in water, with salt, and bring to a boil; simmer 10 to 15 minutes, or until quite tender. Drain thoroughly and chop finely. Add raisins, peanuts, and vinegar; mix well.

To complete the meal, add the ham (a delicatessen slice) and limas (frozen), heated to steaming. (The collards with raisins and peanuts alone contain 100 calories and 6 grams of fiber.)

5

Soups

POTATO SOUP (basic recipe; 3 servings)

Calories per serving: 80   Fiber per serving: 4.5 grams

1   cup diced raw potato (6-ounce potato)
½   cup chopped onion or 2 tablespoons instant minced
     onion
¼   cup minced celery
2   cups chicken broth
     Dash of nutmeg
¼   teaspoon marjoram or thyme
     Salt to taste

Combine all ingredients and cook until potatoes are mushy-soft. Serve yourself ⅓ of the total now; freeze remainder for later. Serve topped with freeze-dried chives or chopped parsley.

POTATO AND SPINACH SOUP

Calories: 120   Fiber: 6 grams

Defrost 1 serving of the basic Potato Soup recipe and purée in blender. Heat with 1 tablespoon bacon-flavored chips and ½ cup chopped raw spinach for about 6 minutes.

POTATO, CHICKEN, AND WATERCRESS SOUP

Calories: 130   Fiber: 5.5 grams

Exactly like Potato and Spinach Soup except add ½ cup minced watercress leaves instead of spinach. Instead of the bacon chips, add 2 tablespoons chopped cooked chicken.

PORTUGUESE POTATO AND BEAN SOUP

Calories: 150   Fiber: 9 grams

Defrost 1 serving of the basic Potato Soup recipe and add ¼ cup cooked or canned kidney beans and 1 tablespoon minced lean ham. Heat.

GARBANZO SOUP

Calories: 150   Fiber: 12.5 grams

¾ cup cooked or canned chickpeas (garbanzos)
¼ cup water
¼ cup grated carrot
2 tablespoons minced celery
   Dash of cayenne pepper or Tabasco sauce
   Dash of garlic salt (optional)
2 tablespoons chopped parsley
1 teaspoon low-fat yogurt

Combine all ingredients except yogurt; purée in blender. Heat. Serve topped with yogurt.

KIDNEY BEAN SOUP (2 portions)

Calories per serving: 120   Fiber per serving: 11 grams

1   cup cooked or canned kidney beans
1   cup canned tomatoes
1   tablespoon minced onion
    Pinch of powdered cloves
    Pinch of rosemary or thyme
2   tablespoons minced parsley

Combine all ingredients except parsley; purée in blender. Simmer 5 to 10 minutes. Serve topped with parsley.

BLACK BEAN SOUP (2 servings)

Calories per serving: 210   Fiber per serving: 19.5 grams

    One 16-ounce can black beans
1   cup water
1   teaspoon minced onion
1   slice lemon
1   tablespoon sherry (optional)

Put beans in the blender, add water, and purée completely. Heat in saucepan; add onion and lemon and simmer 5 minutes. Freeze half the soup for another day; have half now, adding ½ tablespoon sherry.

RED LENTIL SOUP

The little red lentils (which actually are pink) not only do not need presoaking, they cook almost as quickly as rice. You will find them in most health food stores, often sold in bulk.

Calories: 230   Fiber: 8 grams

¼ cup red lentils
1 cup water
½ teaspoon salt
¼ cup chopped carrot
¼ cup chopped apple
½ teaspoon curry powder
   Pinch of cumin (optional)
2 tablespoons nonfat dry milk
⅓ cup water
2 tablespoons Whole-Wheat Croutons

Cook lentils in 1 cup water and salt for 20 minutes. Add carrot, apple, curry powder, and cumin, and cook 10 minutes longer. Dissolve dry milk in ⅓ cup water and stir into lentil mixture. Keep warm but do not allow to simmer after adding milk. Serve topped with croutons.

WHOLE-WHEAT CROUTONS (1½ cups)

Calories per ¼ cup: 30   Fiber per ¼ cup: 1.5 grams

Cut 3 slices of whole-wheat or other whole-grain bread into ½-inch cubes. Spread over a pie pan and slowly toast in oven (300°F.) until crisp and dry, about 25 minutes. Sprinkle with herbs or seasoned salt, or with curry powder, if you like. Put in a plastic bag and seal with a twist tie. Store in a dry place.

BROWN LENTIL SOUP (basic recipe; 4 servings)

Calories per serving: 110   Fiber per serving: 5 grams

⅔ cup dried brown lentils
6   cups chicken broth made with mix
1   lemon, grated, rind and juice
1   clove garlic, crushed
1   cup chopped onions
½   cup chopped carrots
    Pinch of cloves
    Salt and freshly ground black pepper

Combine ingredients, cover, bring just to a simmer, and cook over very low heat about 2 hours. Cool enough to divide into portions for freezing in individual plastic containers with lids.

LENTILS MADRILENA

Calories: 150   Fiber: 9 grams

1   serving basic Brown Lentil Soup
½   cup canned tomatoes, chopped
1   tablespoon chopped green pepper
2   tablespoons grated carrot
2   tablespoons Whole-Wheat Croutons (see page 158)

Combine the soup with tomatoes, green pepper, and carrots; simmer 5 minutes. Serve topped with croutons.

LENTIL SOUP WITH CHEESE

Calories: 160   Fiber: 8 grams

1   serving basic Brown Lentil Soup
1   tablespoon imitation bacon chips
1   tablespoon shredded Swiss cheese

Reheat the soup, adding bacon chips. Put shredded cheese in the bottom of a soup bowl and add the hot soup.

YANKEE BEAN SOUP (2 servings)

Calories per serving: 125   Fiber per serving: 10 grams

1   cup cooked or canned Great Northern beans
½   cup canned tomatoes, chopped
1   envelope beef-flavored broth mix
2   tablespoons grated carrot
1   tablespoon chopped celery leaves
¼   teaspoon thyme or marjoram
2   tablespoons instant minced onion, or chopped fresh onion to taste
Imitation bacon chips

Combine all ingredients but the bacon chips; simmer 10 to 15 minutes, until beans are quite mushy. Have ½ today, save the rest for tomorrow. You may prefer it puréed (in the blender) as a smooth soup. Sprinkle 1 tablespoon bacon chips over each serving.

SPLIT PEA SOUP WITH CROUTONS (basic recipe; 4 servings)

Calories per serving: 65   Fiber per serving: 6 grams

1   cup split green or yellow peas
5   cups water or beef or chicken broth (made with broth mix)
1   cup chopped onion
½   cup chopped celery
1   tablespoon chopped celery leaves
1   teaspoon dried sage or savory
2   tablespoons fresh chopped parsley
    Salt and pepper
    Whole-Wheat Croutons (page 158)

Soak peas overnight in water or broth in a large heavy saucepan. Next day, add remaining ingredients except croutons, bring almost to a boil, lower heat, and simmer 2 hours, or until the peas are soft. (This can be slow-cooked in a crock pot for 8 to 10 hours.) Allow to cool somewhat, then purée in a blender. Divide into servings and freeze 3 of them. Serve each portion topped with croutons.

PEA SOUP WITH HAM

Calories: 130   Fiber: 6 grams

1   serving basic Split Pea Soup
2   tablespoons chopped lean boiled ham
    Whole-Wheat Croutons (page 158)

Reheat the soup, adding ham and croutons.

CHUNKY PEA SOUP

Calories: 160   Fiber: 9.5 grams

1   serving basic Split Pea Soup with Croutons
¼   cup minced or shredded carrots
¼   cup chopped apple
1   tablespoon sunflower kernels

Reheat the soup, adding carrots, apple, and sunflower seed kernels. Bring to a boil and simmer over very low heat 5 to 10 minutes. Serve topped with croutons.

BAKED BEAN SOUP (2 servings)

Calories per serving: 150   Fiber per serving: 9.5 grams

    One 8-ounce can beans with tomato sauce
1   cup canned tomatoes
1   teaspoon instant minced onion, or chopped fresh onion to taste
1   tablespoon imitation bacon bits
½   teaspoon beef-flavored broth mix
    Chili powder to taste
2   tablespoons low-fat yogurt

Combine all ingredients except yogurt, bring to a boil, lower heat, and simmer 10 minutes. Purée in blender. Serve ½ today, save the rest for tomorrow. Top each serving with 1 tablespoon yogurt.

6

Legumes in the F-Plan

Dried beans, peas, and lentils are the highest in fiber count per serving of any foods, and also are high in protein (they're good as meat substitutes) and other important nutrients. Many are available in cans in supermarkets, especially chickpeas, kidney beans, Great Northern (white) beans, and baked beans in several versions. Pinto and black beans can now be found in most supermarkets, having come into popularity as Mexican and Cuban restaurants have sprung up all over the country. Those that top the legume list for fiber content are kidney, pinto, and black beans. Delicious black bean soup is a whiz to prepare—just pour a can of black beans into the blender with added water, purée until smooth, then heat with some instant minced onion or a lemon slice, and you have yourself a meal.

Since you will be eating a lot of legumes on the F-Plan, it may pay you to cook up your favorite dried beans in batches. They will keep well in the refrigerator, and you can take out a cup or ½ cup as needed. To speed presoaking of uncooked dried beans (or peas), put them in water to cover, bring to a boil, simmer just 2 minutes, then turn off the heat and allow to stand 1 hour. Then add more water, and salt, and cook until tender, 2 to 3 hours. Even easier is to use a crock pot: Put beans and water in the pot the night before; next morning, add whatever ingredients are called for in the basic recipe and slow-cook beans (or dried peas) during the day. Long cooking at very low heat does not destroy the fiber, and some beans can be cooked all day. For exact directions, check your crock pot instruction book. Lentils, alone of the dried legumes, do not need presoaking and cook somewhat more quickly than other legumes.

MEALS WITH GOOD OLD BAKED BEANS

There are half a dozen varieties of canned baked beans on supermarket shelves. Before selecting one, be sure to examine the nutritional information on the can to learn the calorie count per serving. This varies greatly from one product to another, from a low of 180 calories per 8-ounce can to 260. The variance is due to the amount of fat, molasses, and sugar added.

FRANKFURTERS AND BEANS

Calories per serving: 215   Fiber per serving: 8 grams

1   frankfurter
½   8-ounce can of baked beans in tomato sauce
     Tomato catsup, mustard, chopped onions to taste

Boil the frankfurter and serve with the beans, catsup, mustard, and onions.

Baked beans on toast are a favorite English snack, and baked bean sandwiches are popular with some Americans, too. Pork and beans, rather than the vegetarian bean version, will make the better sandwich, but be sure to check the calorie count on the can!

BAKED BEAN SANDWICH

Calories: 195   Fiber: 11 grams

¼ cup beans in tomato sauce
1   teaspoon grated fresh onion
1   teaspoon tomato catsup
1   tablespoon shredded carrot
2   slices high-bran bread

Combine all ingredients except bread in blender; purée.
Spread between 2 slices of bread.

BLACK-EYED PEAS SOUTHERN STYLE

Calories: 235   Fiber: 20 grams (with the greens)

1   cup canned or 1 package frozen black-eyed peas
    Dash of garlic powder
1   teaspoon instant minced onion, reconstituted, or
    chopped fresh onion to taste
    Freshly ground black pepper
    Pinch of dried sage or oregano
2   tablespoons chopped lean ham

Combine all ingredients and simmer 10 minutes. Serve
with ½ cup chopped cooked collard greens (fresh or
frozen).

CHICKPEA MEALS

CHICKPEAS WITH PORK

Calories: 375   Fiber: 14 grams

¼ cup lean diced pork (taken from pork chop)
1   teaspoon oil
2   tablespoons chopped onion
1   small tomato, chopped
1   tablespoon chopped green pepper
1   cup chickpeas
1   teaspoon chopped parsley or pinch of dried mint

Put pork with oil and onion in nonstick pan; cook and stir until lightly colored. Add tomato and green pepper, cook 2 minutes longer, then add chickpeas; cook another 3 or 4 minutes. Add parsley or mint just before serving.

GARBANZO SALAD

Calories: 215   Fiber: 13.5 grams

¾ cup canned chickpeas, drained
1   scallion, minced
4   cherry tomatoes, halved
¼ cup chopped green pepper
1   tablespoon minced parsley
1   tablespoon reduced-calorie Italian dressing
2   Ry-Krisps or wheat thins

Combine all ingredients except crackers; toss to blend. Serve with crackers.

GARBANZOS SEVILLANA (2 servings)

Calories per serving: 150   Fiber per serving: 6 grams

¼ cup chopped onion
1 clove garlic, crushed
1 teaspoon oil
½ cup cooked or canned chickpeas
1 small sweet potato, peeled and diced
¼ teaspoon salt
½ cup canned or fresh tomatoes, chopped
½ bay leaf, crushed
1 teaspoon chopped parsley
1 teaspoon imitation bacon chips

Cook onion and garlic in oil in a nonstick pan until softened and lightly colored. Add remaining ingredients except parsley and bacon chips; cook covered, 20 minutes, or until sweet potato is tender. Serve topped with parsley and bacon chips.

KIDNEY BEAN MEALS

CHILI CON CARNE (3 servings)

Calories per serving: 205   Fiber per serving: 7 grams

½   pound lean chopped beef
¼   cup chopped green pepper
¼   cup chopped onion
1   cup cooked or canned kidney beans
1   8-ounce can tomato sauce
½   teaspoon garlic salt
2   teaspoons chili powder
     Cayenne pepper or Tabasco sauce to taste

Put beef, green pepper, and onion in nonstick pan over moderate heat and stir-fry until meat loses its pink color. Drain off fat. Add to remaining ingredients in heavy saucepan and simmer 40 to 45 minutes over low heat. Divide into portions; freeze 2.

KIDNEY BEAN AND PORK CASSEROLE (4 servings)

Calories per serving: 150   Fiber per serving: 7 grams

½   pound lean pork, diced
¼   cup chopped pimento
1   large onion, peeled and chopped
½   cup dried kidney beans (presoaked but not cooked)
1   medium apple, cored and diced
1   cup canned tomatoes
     One 10-ounce can beef consommé diluted with a can of water
     Salt and pepper to taste

Put all ingredients in a large heavy saucepan, bring to a boil, cover, and simmer gently 1½ to 2 hours, until beans are tender. Cook uncovered during last 15 minutes to reduce sauce.

AND MORE LATIN AMERICAN FAVORITES

EASY ENCHILADAS

Calories: 390   Fiber: 14 grams

- 2   corn tortillas
- ½   cup canned or cooked kidney beans
- ¼   cup tomato sauce
- ½   teaspoon chili powder
-         Dash of cayenne pepper
- ¼   teaspoon cumin seeds or ground cumin
- 1   slice salami, chopped
- 2   tablespoons low-fat yogurt

You can buy tortillas frozen or canned; heat them in an ungreased skillet to soften. Heat together the beans, tomato sauce, seasonings, and salami. Put the mixture in the blender for a quick mix, not to purée, but to mash partially. Fill the tortillas, roll up, and place in baking dish. Brush top with yogurt. Bake in 350°F. oven 15 minutes. Add more yogurt over the top when you dish it out.

MEXICAN BEEF AND BEANS (4 servings)

Calories per serving: 170   Fiber per serving: 17 grams

½   pound dried pinto beans
4   cups water
½   pound lean stewing beef in 1-inch cubes
½   teaspoon crushed red pepper flakes
½   cup chopped onion
½   teaspoon garlic salt
2   tablespoons catsup
2   teaspoons chili powder

Soak beans overnight. Next morning add remaining ingredients. Cover and simmer over very low heat until beans are tender, 2 to 3 hours; or slow-cook in a crock pot for 9 hours. Divide into portions; freeze 3 of the 4 portions in plastic containers. Have the remaining portion for your dinner today.

POACHED EGG ON BLACK BEANS

Calories: 275   Fiber: 10.5 grams

1   cup canned or cooked black beans
1   tablespoon minced green pepper
1   tablespoon chopped pimento
1   slice whole-wheat toast
1   large egg
     Salt to taste
     Minced parsley for garnish

Cook beans in a saucepan with green pepper and pimento for 3 or 4 minutes. Spoon onto plate, over a slice of whole-wheat toast. Top with the egg, poached. Sprinkle egg with salt and parsley. (Instead of black beans, both chickpeas and white Great Northern beans can be prepared this way, though the fiber count will not be as high.)

7

Satisfying Hi-Fi Salad Meals

The average salad is not as good a source of fiber (or anything else of much nutritional value) as people imagine. Professor Peter van Soest, one of the top fiber experts in the U.S., has commented that "salad is little more than packaged water." When you combine on your plate a generous quantity of lettuce, cucumber, and radishes, a spring onion, and some watercress, you are unlikely to consume more than 1 gram of dietary fiber.

The salads in this section are especially devised to make a realistic contribution to your daily fiber intake, and at modest calorie cost. You can add other low-calorie vegetables (see page 117).

The calorie cost of salad dressings is not included in the recipes except where it specifically says so. It's the dressing that runs up the calorie total for most salads: A level tablespoon of almost any of the regular commercial dressings contains at least 100 calories. If you make your own dressing with oil and vinegar, the oil costs 100 calories per tablespoon. Mayonnaise, too, has 100 calories in every tablespoon.

We suggest three low-calorie dressings for salads. In addition, there are a number of commercial "reduced-calorie" dressings in the supermarkets, usually to be found in the dietetic section. Before selecting one, be sure to read the nutritional information on the label, where calories per serving is listed. A few have as little as 4 or 6 calories in a tablespoon; others, despite labels that proclaim them to have "less oil, fewer calories," may have as much as 80 or even 90 calories per serving. Some brands in national distribution are suggested; many that may be available in your neighborhood market are not mentioned because their distribution is spotty.

	Calories per tablespoon
Herb Magic Italian Dressing	4
Kraft Zesty Italian Reduced Calorie Dressing	6
Kraft Catalina Reduced Calorie Dressing	16
Reduced Calorie Thousand Island Dressing	20
Wish-Bone Lite Italian	30
Wish-Bone Lite French Style Reduced Calories	30
Kraft Buttermilk Reduced Calorie Dressing	30
Weight Watchers Reduced Calorie Mayonnaise	40
Light 'n' Lively Imitation Mayonnaise (Safeway)	40
Scotch Buy (Safeway) Imitation Mayonnaise	50

Sometimes just a few dashes of olive oil and a sprinkling of lemon juice, along with salt and herbs, will provide all the dressing you need. A teaspoon of olive oil is 33 calories, ½ teaspoon only 17.

Keep in mind that there are 3 teaspoons (level measurement) in each tablespoon, so if you are using just a teaspoon of any of the dressing given above, divide the calorie count by 3.

HOMEMADE LOW-CALORIE SALAD DRESSINGS

TANGY TOMATO DRESSING

Calories: 5   Fiber: 0 grams

1   tablespoon tomato juice
1   teaspoon Worcestershire sauce
1   teaspoon lemon juice or vinegar
     Salt and pepper

Blend all ingredients together.

YOGURT MINT DRESSING

Calories: 10   Fiber: 0 grams

1   tablespoon low-fat natural yogurt
1   teaspoon lemon juice
½   teaspoon chopped fresh mint or ¼ teaspoon
     concentrated mint sauce
     Salt and pepper

Blend all the dressing ingredients together.

TOMATO YOGURT SALAD DRESSING

Calories: 15   Fiber: 0 grams

1   tablespoon tomato juice
1   tablespoon low-fat natural yogurt
     Pinch of sugar
     Pinch of dry mustard
     Salt and pepper

Blend all the dressing ingredients together.

SALAD ENTREES

CHICKEN SALAD WITH CELERY, APPLE, AND WATERCRESS

Calories: 165   Fiber: 5.5 grams

1   small apple, cored and thinly sliced
1   teaspoon lemon juice
1   stalk celery, thinly sliced
5   watercress sprigs
1   slice breast of roast chicken

Toss apple slices with lemon juice; combine with celery and watercress. Remove skin and any fat from the chicken. Put on salad plate, top with salad combination or chopped chicken, and mix with other ingredients. If desired, add a teaspoon of Yogurt Mint Dressing (see page 174), which will increase the calorie count by 10.

FRUIT AND CABBAGE SALAD

Calories: 145   Fiber: 8.5 grams

2   dried apricot halves, chopped
1   tablespoon raisins
2   tablespoons orange juice
½   small crisp red apple
1   tablespoon lemon juice
¼   cup chopped red cabbage
1   celery stalk, chopped

Soak apricots and raisins in orange juice ½ hour. Core and chop apple and toss in lemon juice until coated. Add fruits to cabbage and celery and toss well to mix.

WINTER SALAD

Calories: 160   Fiber: 6 grams

    Pinch of curry powder
1   tablespoon reduced-calorie Italian dressing
¼   red Delicious apple, cored and chopped
2   tablespoons minced celery
2   tablespoons chopped walnuts
2   tablespoons diced white turnip
1   tablespoon chopped green pepper
1   tablespoon raisins

Add curry powder to the dressing; pour dressing over
other ingredients in a bowl and toss to blend. Serve over a
lettuce leaf. (You may also wish to add a teaspoon of
imitation mayonnaise, another 13 calories.)

SCALLOP, ORANGE, AND AVOCADO SALAD

Calories: 200   Fiber: 4 grams

½   seedless orange, peeled and chopped
2   very thin slices onion, broken into rings
2   ounces bay scallops
3   slices avocado
1   tablespoon lemon juice
    Dash of cayenne pepper or crushed red pepper flakes
    Pinch of salt
    Freshly ground black pepper

Remove all white membrane from the orange, then divide
in half and cut 1 half into small pieces with sharp knife,
preserving the juice. (Save the other half for another salad,
or your daily fruit quota.) Put in bowl with the onion
rings, scallops, avocado, lemon juice, and seasonings.

Cover; marinate in refrigerator several hours before serving. (The lemon juice "cooks" the scallops.) Serve this way or over lettuce.

COLESLAW (basic recipe)

Calories: 165   Fiber: 4.5 grams

½   cup shredded green or white cabbage
¼   cup shredded or grated carrots
1   scallion, minced
1   teaspoon reduced-calorie vinaigrette dressing
1   tablespoon low-fat yogurt
    Pinch of dry mustard
2   tablespoons sunflower kernels or chopped peanuts
1   tablespoon minced parsley or dill

Mix cabbage, carrot, and scallion in bowl. Blend dressing, yogurt, and mustard; add to vegetables and mix well. Stir in sunflower kernels or peanuts and parsley.

COLESLAW WITH APPLES AND RAISINS

Calories: 110   Fiber: 5.5 grams

Prepare the basic Coleslaw recipe but add ¼ cup thinly sliced tart apple instead of carrot and 2 tablespoons chopped raisins instead of the nuts.

COLESLAW WITH HAM

Calories: 175   Fiber: 6 grams

Prepare the basic Coleslaw recipe but instead of the sunflower kernels add ⅛ pound diced ham.

COLESLAW WITH CHICKEN AND PEAS

Calories: 170   Fiber: 7 grams

Prepare the basic Coleslaw recipe but add ¼ cup cooked peas (or chopped raw sugar snap peas) in place of the nuts, and add ¼ cup diced cooked chicken as well.

THREE-BEAN SALAD WITH EGG

Calories: 200   Fiber: 8 grams

¼   cup cooked green (snap) beans
¼   cup cooked lima beans
¼   cup cooked or canned kidney beans
2   thin slices onion, in rings
1   tablespoon reduced-calorie vinaigrette dressing
1   hard-cooked egg, sliced
    Lettuce or romaine

Combine the beans with the onion and dressing and marinate 15 minutes. Slice the egg and add to the beans. Serve over lettuce.

ROAST BEEF, CHICKPEA, AND FETA CHEESE SALAD

Calories: 300   Fiber: 8.5 grams

¼   cup minced cooked roast beef
½   cup chickpeas
1   small tomato, chopped
2   tablespoons minced celery
1   teaspoon minced parsley

1   tablespoon reduced-calorie Italian dressing
2   small cubes feta cheese

Combine all ingredients, toss to blend. (Instead of Italian dressing you may prefer Yogurt Mint Dressing, page 174, for this salad.)

SWEDISH POTATO SALAD

Calories: 235   Fiber: 8 grams

1   small potato, boiled and diced
1   teaspoon olive oil
   Salt
½   small tart apple, cored and thinly sliced
1   scallion, chopped
1   teaspoon minced parsley or dill
   Sprinkling of caraway seeds
1   teaspoon vinegar
2   small whole beets, cooked

While potato is still warm, toss with oil and sprinkle with salt. Add apple, scallion, parsley or dill, caraway seeds, and vinegar. Mix well. Cover; chill. Put on salad plate with the beets.

BEET, CARROT, AND SHRIMP SALAD

Calories: 95   Fiber: 5 grams

1   tablespoon low-fat yogurt
1   teaspoon horseradish
¼   cup sliced cooked beets
⅓   cup diced scraped carrot
¼   cup canned or frozen cooked shrimp, drained
⅓   cup bean sprouts
5   watercress sprigs

Combine yogurt and horseradish, add to beets, carrot, and shrimp in bowl, and stir to blend. Serve garnished with bean sprouts and watercress.

COOKED VEGETABLE SALAD

Calories: 130   Fiber: 8 grams

⅓   cup diced cooked potato
2   small broccoli spears, cooked
¼   cup sliced cooked beets
1   tablespoon reduced-calorie vinaigrette dressing

Arrange vegetables on plate; add dressing.

Another possible salad combination: ⅓ cup potato, ½ cup cooked carrot, and ½ cup cooked green beans or Italian beans. This would be 100 calories and 6 grams of fiber.

For more protein, a sliced hard-cooked egg could be added, for another 80 calories—but no additional fiber.

MIXED VEGETABLE AND CHEESE SALAD

Calories: 125   Fiber: 5 grams

3	thin slices of raw cauliflower sprigs
¼	cup cooked green peas
1	tablespoon chopped green pepper
1	ounce Edam cheese, cut into tiny cubes or grated
1	tablespoon reduced-calorie Italian dressing
	Salt and pepper to taste

Combine all ingredients and toss to blend with dressing.

TABOULEH (Lebanese wheat salad)

Calories: 110   Fiber: 8 grams

¼	cup fine bulgur
2	tablespoons minced green pepper
1	scallion, minced
½	small tomato, seeded and chopped
1	tablespoon minced parsley
1	teaspoon lemon juice
1	tablespoon salad oil
	Salt and pepper to taste
8	lettuce leaves

Put bulgur in bowl, add water to cover, let stand until most of liquid is absorbed, then press through a sieve to remove any remaining liquid. Combine with all remaining ingredients but the lettuce leaves; chill. To serve, spoon the salad mixture into lettuce leaves, roll up, and eat with fingers. (It can be served over shredded lettuce, but somehow it tastes much better the other way.)

SHRIMP AND PEPPER SALAD

Calories: 100   Fiber: 4 grams

½   green pepper, seeded and chopped
½   cup bean sprouts
1   small tomato, quartered
2   ounces (⅓ of 6-ounce package) frozen small shrimp, cooked
¼   teaspoon curry powder
¼   teaspoon basil
     Salt
1   tablespoon lemon juice

Combine all ingredients. Yogurt Mint Dressing (page 174) is very nice with this; if you use it, add 10 calories to the total.

See also Garbanzo Salad (page 166) and "Salads to Accompany Meals" (see following page).

8

Salads to Accompany Meals

CRESS, CUCUMBER, AND TOMATO SALAD

Calories: 30   Fiber: 3 grams

½   small tomato, sliced
1   scallion, minced
1   tablespoon reduced-calorie Italian dressing
½   cup watercress, leaves only
¼   cup thinly sliced cucumber
¼   cup bean sprouts

Combine tomato and scallion in bowl, add dressing, and let stand at least 15 minutes before adding cress, cucumber, and bean sprouts.

SALADE RUSSE

Calories: 75   Fiber: 11 grams

½   package frozen peas and carrots, cooked
¼   cup minced celery
2   tablespoons cooked or canned Great Northern beans
1   teaspoon imitation mayonnaise
1   teaspoon reduced-calorie vinaigrette dressing

Combine peas and carrots, celery, and beans. Toss with imitation mayonnaise, then vinaigrette dressing.

TOMATO-ZUCCHINI SALAD

Calories: 60   Fiber: 3 grams

1   small ripe tomato, sliced
¼   cup zucchini, thinly sliced
¼   teaspoon chervil or tarragon
      Salt to taste
1   teaspoon olive oil

Arrange tomato and zucchini slices on plate and sprinkle with herb and salt, then oil. Let stand awhile before eating.

ITALIAN WHITE BEAN SALAD

Calories: 85   Fiber: 8.5 grams

½   cup cooked or canned Great Northern beans
2   tablespoons chopped parsley
1   teaspoon grated onion, or 1 scallion, minced
      Dash of vinegar
1   teaspoon Italian herb seasoning

Combine ingredients. Chill before serving.

MARINATED CARROT SALAD

Calories: 55   Fiber: 4 grams

½   cup sliced carrots
2   tablespoons minced parsley
1   teaspoon olive oil
½   teaspoon vinegar
      Salt to taste

Cook carrots in a small amount of water just until barely tender, still a little crisp, about 4 minutes. Drain. While they are still warm, add parsley and oil. Later add vinegar and salt. Chill.

9

Hi-Fi Pizzas, Muffins, and Pancakes

Americans have a love affair with pizza that's almost un-
believable. One can understand why the young like hand-
to-mouth eating, but pizza appears to have no age limit,
and pizza gourmets delight in using wildly imaginative
toppings.

When pizza is made with whole-wheat flour, with some
bran thrown in for good measure, it becomes an excellent
fiber source, with just the standard tomato sauce and
cheese topping. When the topping ingredients also are
fiber-rich and imaginative, you have something great.

For those who enjoy getting their hands on a ball of
yeast dough, pizza can be made at home, simplified by a
food processor. Then you can make individual pizza
shells, freeze them, and have them ready for meals any-
time. Or you can, of course, make a full-size pizza and cut
it into portions before freezing, then wrap each portion
separately.

We give you a basic pizza crust recipe, sauce, and four
toppings in measurements for single portions. These are
good-sized single-serving shells, equivalent to having two
slices of bread, fiber-wise.

And if you aren't up to making your own, a shortcut
version is whole-wheat English muffins. Not all markets
carry these, and some brands are much tastier than others.
They are more available, and better, on the West Coast
than in other parts of the country. If you can find them,
and like those you find, here is how to turn them into
pizza shells: Split open with a fork, press the center down
a little, to hold the topping, then divide the ingredients for
single servings over the 2 halves and place under the

broiler, rather than in the oven, as for regular crusts.

Much easier to make than pizza dough are muffins, which can be stirred up in a minute or two. These, too, can be wrapped in serving portions (2 in a bag) to freeze and store.

PIZZAS

HI-FI PIZZA (basic recipe; 8 servings)

Calories per serving: 175   Fiber per serving: 6.5 grams

1   envelope active dry yeast
1   teaspoon salt
1   cup warm (120°F.) water
2   tablespoons oil
2⅔ cups unsifted whole-wheat flour
¼   cup bran
⅓   cup rolled oats

Dissolve yeast and salt in warm water (try a drop on your wrist; it should feel lukewarm). Add the oil, then gradually beat in half the flour. (If you have a food processor, you can add it all at once and let the processor blades do the beating.) Beat in the bran and oats, then the rest of the flour, until you have a stiff but pliable dough that comes away from the side of the bowl and can be lifted in one piece. Turn out on board, knead about 3 minutes, then put into a greased mixing bowl, turning to grease on all sides. Cover, let rise in warm place until doubled in bulk, then remove to shape.

This recipe will make 2 regular full-size pizzas, or 1 full-size and 4 single-serving pizzas, or 8 individual pizzas. If you want to make one for the family (or to serve guests) while you are in the pizza-making mood, divide dough in half; form 4 balls of equal size with the first half and 1 large ball with the second part. Fit the large half over a pizza pan, making it thicker around the edges. With the rest, press out each ball of dough into a circle, using fingers and the heel of your palm, somewhat higher around the edge than in the center. Or make 8 balls and form individual shells.

You can add the topping *before* freezing, if you like—all but the cheese, which should be added just before you pop the pizza into the oven. Or you can freeze the crusts, and add the topping on them later. Place in the freezer, on a baking sheet, until frozen hard, then remove and wrap individually in plastic wrap or foil and return to freezer.

To bake, with the topping and cheese added, preheat oven to 400°F. and bake 20 to 25 minutes, for a full-size pizza. For individual pizzas, baking time is reduced to 10 to 15 minutes, or until cheese is melted, the filling sizzling, and the crust golden.

PIZZA SAUCE (basic recipe; 16 servings)

Calories per serving: 10   Fiber per serving: 0.5 gram

    One 16-ounce can tomato sauce
1   teaspoon olive oil
1   or 2 cloves garlic, crushed, or 1 teaspoon garlic powder
½   cup chopped onion
½   teaspoon oregano
1   tablespoon parsley

Combine all ingredients; simmer 15 minutes. One cup of sauce may be frozen: Pour into pint jar and allow ample headroom for expansion when freezing. Keep the second half in the refrigerator, to use as needed. For single servings, use 2 tablespoons sauce; for 1 large pizza, ½ cup sauce. Add 2 tablespoons grated cheese per serving, or a 1-ounce slice of cheese (Swiss, mozzarella, Cheddar, or American) cut to fit.

Toppings for Individual Pizzas

ZUCCHINI SHRIMP PIZZA

Calories: 260   Fiber: 8 grams

¼ cup thinly sliced zucchini
2 ounces (⅓ of a 6-ounce package) frozen tiny shrimp
1 tablespoon bean sprouts
1 individual pizza shell
  Salt to taste
½ teaspoon basil or marjoram
1 teaspoon diet margarine
1 tablespoon shredded Swiss cheese

Arrange zucchini, shrimp, and bean sprouts over pizza. Sprinkle with salt and herb, dot with margarine, then top with cheese. Bake in preheated 400°F. oven for 10 or 15 minutes, until crust is golden and cheese melted.

ARTICHOKE PIZZA

Calories: 275   Fiber: 11 grams

3   canned artichoke hearts (water-packed), coarsely chopped
1   scallion, minced
1   tablespoon chopped pimento
1   individual pizza shell
½   teaspoon Italian herb seasoning mix
2   tablespoons Pizza Sauce (page 188)
2   black olives, sliced
1   thin slice mozzarella cheese, cut to fit

Arrange artichokes, scallion, and pimento over pizza. Sprinkle with herbs, then spread with sauce. Add olives. Put cheese on top. Bake in preheated 400°F. oven for 10 minutes, until crust is golden and cheese melted.

FRESH TOMATO PIZZA WITH MUSHROOMS

Calories: 235   Fiber: 8.5 grams

¼   cup sliced mushrooms
1   individual pizza shell
    Salt and pepper to taste
¼   teaspoon mixed herbs (basil, oregano, parsley)
2   tomato slices
1   thin slice mozzarella or Swiss cheese

Arrange mushrooms over pizza; sprinkle with salt and herbs; add tomato slices, cut to fit over mushrooms; sprinkle tomato with salt, pepper, and herbs. Cover with cheese. Bake in 400°F. oven 10 to 15 minutes, until cheese is melted and tomato softened.

CHILI CON CARNE PIZZA

Calories: 355   Fiber: 11 grams

2   tablespoons chopped beef
1   tablespoon chopped chili pepper, red or green
½   teaspoon chili powder
    Dash of cayenne pepper
    Garlic salt to taste
2   tablespoons canned kidney beans
1   individual pizza shell
2   tablespoons Pizza Sauce (page 188)
2   tablespoons grated Cheddar cheese

Cook beef and chili pepper together in nonstick pan, stirring, until meat loses its pink color; pour off accumulated fat. Add chili powder, cayenne, and garlic salt; stir to blend. Add beans. Spoon over pizza; top with sauce and then grated cheese. Bake in 400°F. oven for 10 to 15 minutes, until crust is golden and cheese melted and sizzling.

Muffins

RAISIN BRAN MUFFINS (makes 12)

Calories (2 muffins): 170   Fiber (2 muffins): 6 grams

1¾ cups unsifted whole-wheat flour
¼ cup bran
½ teaspoon salt
2 teaspoons baking powder
1 tablespoon grated lemon rind
1 egg
1 tablespoon diet margarine
½ cup skim milk
½ cup shredded carrots
¼ cup chopped raisins

Combine everything in mixing bowl; stir just to moisten flour completely. Spoon into 12 nonstick or paper-lined muffin cups. Bake in preheated 400°F. oven for 20 minutes, or until muffins pull away from sides.

ZUCCHINI NUT MUFFINS (makes 12)

Calories (2 muffins): 160   Fiber (2 muffins): 5 grams

1¾ cups unsifted whole-wheat flour
⅓ cup rolled oats
½ teaspoon salt
2 teaspoons baking powder
1 egg
1 tablespoon diet margarine
½ cup skim milk
½ cup finely shredded zucchini
¼ cup chopped sliced almonds

Combine ingredients in a bowl; stir just to moisten flour and oats completely. Spoon into 12 nonstick or paper-lined muffin cups. Bake in preheated 400°F. oven for 20 minutes, or until muffins pull away from sides.

PANCAKES

If you become hungry for pancakes, don't worry. They can make a fine fiber-rich supper, if they are made with whole-grain flours or cornmeal. You must limit yourself to 2 four-inch pancakes, and no butter or syrup, but you can spread them with low-fat cottage cheese, raspberry jam, or cranberry sauce or relish.

WHOLE-WHEAT PANCAKES (makes 2 four-inch pancakes)

Calories: 270   Fiber: 4 grams

¼   cup whole-wheat flour
¼   teaspoon baking powder
     Pinch of salt
1   teaspoon diet margarine
3   to 4 tablespoons skim milk
1   small egg
2   tablespoons cranberry sauce

Blend together flour, baking powder, and salt, without sifting. Beat in margarine, milk, and egg just until flour is completely moistened. Bake on hot nonstick griddle, or one barely moistened with fat (rub surface with brown paper touched with fat). Top with cranberry sauce.

MIXED-GRAIN PANCAKES (makes 2 four-inch pancakes)

Calories: 255   Fiber: 4 grams

Prepare just like Whole-Wheat Pancakes except that instead of ¼ cup whole-wheat flour, use 3 tablespoons whole-wheat flour, ½ tablespoon bran, and 1 tablespoon rolled oats. Instead of cranberry sauce, spread with 2 tablespoons low-fat cottage cheese.

CORNMEAL PANCAKES

Calories (2 thick cakes): 460   Fiber (2 thick cakes): 8 grams

¼   cup stone-ground cornmeal or masa harina
¼   cup whole-wheat flour
½   teaspoon baking powder
     Pinch of salt
1   tablespoon diet margarine
⅓   cup buttermilk
1   egg
2   tablespoons cranberry-orange relish

Blend together in mixing bowl the cornmeal, flour, baking powder, and salt. Make a well in the center and add margarine, buttermilk, and egg. Beat just to moisten the flour and beat in margarine. Bake on nonstick griddle or one barely moistened with fat (rubbed on with brown paper touched with fat). Serve spread with relish.

10

Easy Whole-Grain Pilafs

There are several whole-grain cereals, available in health-food stores, that are excellent fiber sources and can be combined with other ingredients for meal-in-one entrees. Bulgur is probably the best-known; this is cracked whole wheat, much used in the Middle East. Buckwheat groats, better known as kasha, is a great Eastern European favorite. The cereal grain that most people think of first when the word "pilaf" is mentioned is rice, and brown rice is recommended, though lower in fiber than bulgur or buckwheat.

BULGUR PILAF (basic recipe)

Calories: 275   Fiber: 14 grams

- ⅓   cup fine-grain bulgur
- ½   teaspoon salt
- 2   tablespoons chopped carrot
- 2   tablespoons chopped raisins
- 1   tablespoon sunflower kernels
- ⅔   cup boiling water

Put first five ingredients in a saucepan, add the water, bring again to a boil, and simmer, covered, until all liquid is absorbed, about 12 minutes.

BULGUR PILAF WITH BROILED SCROD

Calories: 480   Fiber: 18 grams

⅓ cup fine-grain bulgur
¼ cup frozen tiny green peas, or cooked lima beans
1 4-ounce piece of scrod
2 tablespoons yogurt
   Salt
   Paprika

Prepare Bulgur Pilaf as in the basic recipe, but instead of carrots, add the frozen tiny green peas, or cooked lima beans. Arrange the piece of scrod in the broiler oven (first lining the pan with foil) and spread with the yogurt. Sprinkle with salt and paprika. Broil, on one side only, about 10 minutes, or just until fish flakes easily.

BULGUR PILAF WITH CHICKEN

Calories: 435   Fiber: 14 grams

Prepare Bulgur Pilaf as in the basic recipe but add ½ cup chopped cooked chicken, with all skin and fat removed.

KASHA WITH BEEF (OR PORK) AND BROCCOLI

Calories: 390   Fiber: 10 grams

¼ cup chopped scallions
1 teaspoon diet margarine
⅓ cup buckwheat groats
1 package beef-flavored broth mix

¼   cup chopped cooked beef or pork (leftover)
⅔   cup boiling water
2   broccoli spears

Stir-fry scallions in margarine until lightly colored; do not allow to burn. Combine with the buckwheat groats, broth mix, and meat in a saucepan. Add the boiling water. Bring to a boil, lower heat, and cook, covered, at very low heat for 20 to 30 minutes. During last 5 minutes, cook the broccoli spears in boiling salted water, just until they can be pierced with a fork.

BROWN RICE PILAF WITH LIMAS (2 servings)

Calories per serving: 115   Fiber per serving: 5.5 grams

1¼   cups water
½   teaspoon salt
2   tablespoons chopped celery
1   teaspoon instant minced onion
½   cup brown rice, rinsed and drained
2   apricot halves, chopped
⅓   package frozen baby or Fordhook limas

Bring water to a boil with salt, celery, and onion; add the rice, then apricot and limas. Cover and cook over lowest heat 35 to 40 minutes, until all water is absorbed and there are holes in the rice.

11

Whole-Wheat Pastas

Pasta made with whole-wheat flour has several times as much fiber as that made with refined white flour, and spinach noodles made with whole wheat are even better. Whole-wheat pasta can be found in health food stores and in many gourmet food shops.

MINESTRONE (3 servings)

Calories per serving: 170   Fiber per serving: 11 grams

    One 10-ounce package frozen peas and carrots
2   tablespoons chopped celery
1   cup canned tomatoes, chopped
½   cup canned or cooked Great Northern beans
1   tablespoon instant minced onion or ¼ cup chopped fresh onion
⅛   pound (¼ of 8-ounce package) whole-wheat elbow macaroni (or long macaroni broken in bits)
¼   teaspoon oregano
½   teaspoon thyme or Italian herb seasoning mix
1   cup beef broth
½   cup shredded white cabbage
3   teaspoons chopped fresh parsley
3   teaspoons grated Parmesan cheese
    Salt to taste

Combine peas and carrots, celery, tomatoes, beans, onion, macaroni, and herbs in 2-quart saucepan. Add beef broth. Bring to a boil and cook 10 minutes, or until macaroni is tender. Add cabbage; cook until cabbage is soft. Serve yourself one-third today; store the rest for other meals. Serve topped with parsley and cheese.

SPINACH LASAGNE (2 servings)

Calories per serving: 215   Fiber per serving: 6.5 grams

¼ pound (half of 8-ounce package) whole-wheat lasagne
1 teaspoon diet margarine
¼ cup chopped onion
2 tablespoons chopped parsley
¼ teaspoon oregano or basil
½ 10-ounce package frozen chopped spinach
4 tablespoons ricotta cheese
2 tablespoons skim milk or low-fat yogurt
1 cup (8-ounce can) tomato sauce
 Dash of garlic salt
3 tablespoons Parmesan cheese

Cook the lasagne, rinse and drain under cold water. Melt margarine in nonstick pan, add onion, parsley and oregano; stir-fry until onion is lightly colored. Add spinach, break up with fork. Arrange half the lasagne in 2-quart freeze-and-bake casserole, add spinach mixture, then spread over the spinach the cottage cheese blended with milk or yogurt. Add remaining lasagne. Sprinkle garlic salt into tomato sauce, pour over lasagne. Top with Parmesan cheese. Bake in 400°F. oven until top is browned and sauce bubbling. Remove half for today's portion; keep the rest in the dish, cover, and keep until tomorrow to reheat. Or the remaining half when cool can be transferred to foil and wrapped in a packet for freezing.

SPAGHETTI BOLOGNESE

Calories: 370   Fiber: 14 grams

¼   cup extra-lean chopped beef
¼   cup minced onion
¼   cup minced celery
1   teaspoon instant beef-flavored broth mix
½   cup puréed canned tomato, or tomato sauce
    Pinch of Italian herb seasoning
¼   cup frozen peas
⅛   pound (¼ of 8-ounce package) whole-wheat spaghetti

Make the sauce first: Cook beef in nonstick pan, stirring until it has lost its color. Drain off fat. Add onion, celery, broth mix, tomato, and herbs. Simmer gently 30 to 40 minutes, stirring occasionally. Add water if it cooks down too much. During last 5 minutes, add peas. Meantime, cook spaghetti in rapidly boiling water to *al dente,* about 8 to 10 minutes; drain. Arrange spaghetti on serving platter; cover with the sauce.

WHOLE-WHEAT PASTA WITH CHICKEN LIVERS

Calories: 415   Fiber: 8 grams

¼   pound chicken livers, cut in pieces
1   teaspoon diet margarine
¼   cup sliced mushrooms
    Pinch of oregano
½   cup tomato sauce
1   teaspoon beef broth flavoring
1   tablespoon dry sherry
⅛   pound (¼ of 8-ounce package) whole-wheat linguine
    or spaghetti

Put chicken livers in nonstick pan with margarine and cook until lightly browned. Add mushrooms and cook 3 minutes longer. Add oregano, tomato sauce, and beef broth flavoring. Simmer 15 minutes. (If a thicker sauce is preferred, cook longer to reduce volume.) Stir in sherry.

Meantime, cook pasta in rapidly boiling salted water just until *al dente,* about 8 to 10 minutes. Drain thoroughly and serve topped with livers and sauce.

WHOLE-WHEAT SPAGHETTI WITH RED CLAM SAUCE (2 servings)

Calories per serving: 320   Fiber per serving: 7.5 grams

One 8-ounce can tomato sauce
One 7-ounce can minced clams and liquid
Pinch of oregano or Italian herb seasoning
1   tablespoon instant minced onion, or chopped fresh onion to taste
1   tablespoon grated carrot
Dash of garlic salt or powder
⅛   pound (¼ of 8-ounce package) whole-wheat spaghetti (for 1 serving)

Combine tomato sauce, clams and liquid, oregano, onion, carrot, and garlic salt. Simmer 10 minutes. Cook the spaghetti and serve with half the sauce.

CHICKEN NOODLE CASSEROLE

Calories: 415   Fiber: 8.5 grams

1   cup whole-wheat spinach egg noodles
½   teaspoon diet margarine
4   large mushrooms, sliced
     Salt
¼   teaspoon rosemary
¼   teaspoon thyme or chervil
1   tablespoon whole-wheat flour
½   cup skim milk
½   cup leftover cooked chicken, cut in pieces
¼   teaspoon salt
     Dash of nutmeg
     Paprika

Cook noodles in boiling salted water 8 to 10 minutes; drain thoroughly. Melt margarine in nonstick pan, add mushrooms, sprinkle with salt and herbs, and stir-cook until lightly colored. Add flour, blend well, and gradually stir in milk. Cook until thickened and smooth. Add chicken and seasoning; simmer 5 minutes. Arrange cooked noodles like nest on plate and spoon chicken in center.

12

Between-Meal Light Snacks

When you have calories to spare, these snacks can be enjoyed between meals.

GRAHAM CRACKER EGGNOG

Calories: 270   Fiber: 3 grams

4   graham crackers
1   cup skim milk
1   small egg
1   teaspoon vanilla extract

Combine ingredients in blender and process until foamy.

ARTICHOKE DIP WITH WHEAT THINS

Calories: 80   Fiber: 3.5 grams

4   canned water-packed artichoke hearts, well drained
1   tablespoon imitation mayonnaise
1   teaspoon sesame seeds
    Garlic powder or other seasoning to taste
4   Wheat Thins

Chop the artichoke hearts coarsely with sharp knife. Put all ingredients except Wheat Thins in blender and process until reasonably smooth. Spread 1 tablespoon of the dip on each cracker (¼ cup of dip altogether).

HUMUS DIP FOR VEGETABLES
(approximately 10 dip servings)

Calories per serving for dip: 30
Fiber per serving for dip: 1 gram

1   cup canned chickpeas, drained
1   tablespoon olive oil
2   tablespoons minced parsley
    Garlic powder to taste
    Dash of cayenne pepper or Tabasco sauce
2   tablespoons low-fat yogurt

Put chickpeas, oil, parsley, and seasonings in blender with yogurt. Purée until smooth. Serve as a dip, allowing yourself no more than 2 tablespoons altogether.

Suggested vegetables to be served with the humus: mushrooms, cauliflower buds, carrot sticks, zucchini slivers, and green or red pepper sticks. Black olives are traditionally served as garnish. (For calorie and fiber count of these vegetables, see chart, page 61.)

MEXICAN BEAN DIP

Calories per serving: 115   Fiber per serving: 5 grams

¼   cup canned dark red kidney beans, drained; reserve 1
    tablespoon bean liquid
½   teaspoon chili powder
    Dash of cayenne pepper or Tabasco sauce
½   teaspoon cumin
4   Tostitos (tortilla) chips

Put reserved bean liquid in blender. Measure out ¼ cup of the beans, add to blender with seasonings, and process until puréed. Serve with chips. (We recommend Tostitos because they are made with stone-ground cornmeal, but they are high in fat and salt, so go slow!)

There is one thing wrong with this as a snack: It will take enormous discipline to limit yourself to just 4 filled chips.

POPCORN

Calories per cup: 20   Fiber per cup: 1 gram

If you can enjoy popped corn popped in a hot-air popper, without any fat added—no butter or margarine—this makes a fine high-fiber snack. A little salt is permitted. Serve with Tab or Diet Pepsi.

BUTTERMILK AND GRAHAM CRACKERS

Calories: 135   Fiber: 1.5 grams

Allow yourself 2 graham crackers with one 8-ounce glass chilled buttermilk as a bedtime snack.

13

Hi-Fi Low-Cal Desserts

Since you must have fruit every day as part of the F-Plan program, whole fresh fruit makes the best dessert—lowest in calories, highest in fiber per portion. But if "made" desserts appeal to you more, and you feel a meal just isn't finished without a bit of something sweet at the end, here are some suggestions, each fiber-rich but reasonably low in calories. Add only if your daily quota permits, of course.

STRAWBERRY-ORANGE COMPOTE

Calories: 60   Fiber: 2.5 grams

½   cup strawberries, sliced
½   small orange

Put strawberries in a dessert dish. Carefully peel the orange, removing every bit of white membrane; slice, then cut in smaller pieces into the same dish to save all the juice.

BLACKBERRIES TOPPED WITH YOGURT

Calories: 125   Fiber: 10 grams

1   cup canned blackberries, drained
1   teaspoon lemon juice
2   tablespoons low-fat yogurt

Sprinkle berries with lemon juice to make the flavor more

piquant. Serve topped with yogurt. (If using fresh berries, sprinkle with 1 teaspoon sugar, which adds 16 calories.)

RASPBERRY-BANANA GELATIN (6 servings)

Calories per serving: 55   Fiber per serving: 3 grams

One 3-ounce package fruit-flavored gelatin
1½ cups hot water
1   teaspoon lemon juice
    One 10-ounce package frozen raspberries
½   cup sliced bananas
¼   cup chopped walnuts

Put gelatin in bowl, add hot water, and stir to dissolve. Add lemon juice and frozen raspberries, right out of the package; stir until fruit is completely separated and gelatin has started to set. Stir in bananas and nuts. Pour into 6 individual ¾-cup molds. This will give you desserts for 6 meals, on days when your quota will allow just 55 additional calories.

AMBROSIA

Calories: 110   Fiber: 6 grams

½   small orange
½   banana, sliced
1   tablespoon dried coconut

Peel the orange carefully, removing all white membrane. Cut into dessert dish to preserve all juice. Add bananas and coconut. Stir to mix well; chill.

STRAWBERRIES WITH ALMONDS AND YOGURT

Calories: 100   Fiber: 4 grams

1   cup sliced strawberries
1   teaspoon sugar
1   tablespoon sliced almonds
1   tablespoon low-fat yogurt

Sprinkle strawberries with sugar; chill for 15 or 20 minutes. Chop the sliced almonds and add to the yogurt. Spoon yogurt over berries.

STRAWBERRY-APPLE-APRICOT GELATIN
(6 servings)

Calories per serving: 75   Fiber per serving: 5 grams

½   red Delicious apple, thinly sliced
1   teaspoon lemon juice
     One 3-ounce package lemon-flavored gelatin
1   cup hot water
12 large ice cubes
½   cup sliced strawberries
6   dried apricots, softened in hot water, chopped
3   tablespoons walnuts

Slice apple and sprinkle slices with lemon juice. Dissolve gelatin in hot water; add ice cubes, and stir until most ice has melted and gelatin begins to set. Remove remaining ice. Add fruit and nuts. Spoon into 6 individual ¾-cup molds and chill until firm.

CRANBERRY-ORANGE-DATE SALAD (2 servings)

Calories per serving: 75   Fiber per serving: 2.5 grams

¼ cup chopped raw cranberries
1   small orange, peeled and chopped
2   pitted dates, chopped
2   tablespoons honey

Make sure all white membrane is removed from the orange before cutting it up, then combine the ingredients. Divide into 2 portions and have half today. The rest gets even better as it marinates.

APRICOT-GRAPE COMPOTE

Calories: 110   Fiber: 2.5 grams

2   canned apricot halves or 1 large fresh apricot, pitted, cut in half
10 white grapes
1   teaspoon dried coconut

Combine and chill.

CANNED APRICOTS WITH YOGURT

Calories: 100   Fiber: 2.5 grams

3   canned apricot halves, drained
2   tablespoons low-fat yogurt

Put apricot halves in dessert dish and top with yogurt.

STRAWBERRY-PEACH-APPLE SALAD

Calories: 85   Fiber: 4 grams

¼   pint (½ cup) strawberries, sliced
½   small apple, peeled, cored, and sliced
½   fresh peach, peeled and chopped
      Few drops lemon juice
1   teaspoon sugar

Combine all ingredients and chill about 30 minutes before serving.

FRESH PEACHES WITH YOGURT

Calories: 70   Fiber: 2.5 grams

1   medium peach, peeled, pitted, and sliced
1   teaspoon sugar
      Dash of cinnamon
2   tablespoons low-fat yogurt

Sprinkle peach slices with sugar and cinnamon; top with yogurt. (With 2 canned peach halves, omit the sugar; sprinkle with lemon juice and cinnamon. Because they are put up in syrup, the calorie count will be higher, so add another 30 calories.)

PEAR-PEACH COMPOTE (4 servings)

Calories per serving: 80   Fiber per serving: 3 grams

2   large pears
2   medium peaches
¼   cup sugar

1   lemon, cut in half
1   cup water

Scald the pears and peaches with boiling water to remove skins easily. Put whole fruit in saucepan (or cut each in half and remove cores and pits). Add sugar, lemon, and water; bring to a boil and simmer until largest fruit is fork-tender. Chill in the syrup. Serve yourself 1 whole fruit or 2 halves (without the syrup) for each dessert.

LOW-CALORIE APPLESAUCE (basic recipe; 4 servings)

Calories per serving: 100   Fiber per serving: 4.5 grams

4   large McIntosh apples, cored and quartered
    Sliver of lemon rind
    Pinch of cloves
¼   cup water
2   tablespoons sugar

Put apples in saucepan with lemon rind, cloves, and water; cook until apples are soft enough to mash. Drain off any excess liquid. Stir in sugar. Divide into portions. Chill. (Some people like the peel left on the apple, and the peel is important for fiber.)

APPLESAUCE WITH ALMONDS AND YOGURT

Calories: 120   Fiber: 5 grams

1   serving Low-Calorie Applesauce
1   tablespoon sliced almonds
1   tablespoon low-fat yogurt

Combine and blend lightly.

APPLESAUCE WITH RAISINS

Calories: 130   Fiber: 5.5 grams

1   serving Low-Calorie Applesauce
1   tablespoon raisins
    Dash of cinnamon

Combine and stir to blend well.

BANANA-PEACH DESSERT

Calories: 100   Fiber: 3.5 grams

½   medium banana, sliced
1   small peach, peeled and chopped
1   teaspoon lemon juice
    Grated lemon rind
1   teaspoon sugar

Put banana and peach in dessert dish, sprinkle with lemon juice and rind, then add sugar and blend well. Chill.

BAKED APPLE (basic recipe)

Calories: 95   Fiber: 4.5 grams

1   large baking apple
1   teaspoon honey or brown sugar

Wash apple and remove core with an apple corer or small sharp knife, getting out all seeds. Then cut through apple skin around the center of the apple to prevent it bursting when it bakes. Put in small ovenproof dish, pour 2 tablespoons water around it, and sprinkle top with honey or sugar. Bake at 350°F. for 30 to 40 minutes, until apple is tender and about to grow out of its skin. Serve hot or cold.

BAKED APPLE STUFFED WITH RAISINS AND NUTS

Calories: 155   Fiber: 6 grams

Prepare as in Baked Apple but omit honey or sugar; instead, fill the core with 1 tablespoon chopped raisins and 1 teaspoon chopped walnuts.

BAKED APPLE STUFFED WITH MIXED DRIED FRUIT

Calories: 155   Fiber: 8.5 grams

Prepare as in Baked Apple but omit honey or sugar; instead, fill the core with 1 dried apricot half, 1 pitted prune, and 1 pitted date, all chopped.

RASPBERRY YOGURT

Calories: 105   Fiber: 2.5 grams

¼ cup raspberries, fresh, or frozen and thawed
2   teaspoons confectioner's sugar
½ cup low-fat yogurt

Crush raspberries with sugar and beat in yogurt. Chill before serving.

BLACKBERRY YOGURT

Calories: 80   Fiber: 3 grams

⅓   cup fresh or canned blackberries
½   cup low-fat yogurt

If fresh berries are used (if you are lucky enough to find them at a roadside market, or in the woods), add 2 teaspoons confectioner's sugar and mash the berries well before adding the yogurt. Canned blackberries are soft enough to blend easily; no additional sugar is necessary.

14

Some Sample Daily Menus

Here we show examples of the ways F-Plan meals can be put together to suit your own way of life and preferred eating pattern.

As you follow the diet program you will probably, if you are typical of most dieters, keep returning to some favorite meals that you will learn by heart. But do sample new dishes as well to keep your diet interesting and nutritious.

It is impossible to come up with an exact count of 1,000 or 1,250 (or whatever quota you have decided on) each day, but, using a pocket calculator as you select dishes and menus that appeal to you, try to make the daily total as close to the goal as possible, and if you run over one day, keep it under the next, by the same approximate count.

If you prefer to do so, you can, of course, have all your Fiber-Filler at one time instead of dividing it into two portions—but you must finish it all everyday.

1,000-Calorie Menu for a Working Woman

This suggests a daily meal pattern for a woman who plans to take her lunch to work with her and wants something quick and easy to prepare when she comes home.

	Calories	Grams of Fiber
Daily Allowance:		
Fiber-Filler, 1 cup skim milk, 2 pieces of fruit	400	20
Breakfast		
Half portion of Fiber-Filler with milk from allowance		
Orange from allowance		
Carry-Out Lunch		
Peanut Butter and Jam Sandwich (page 134)	290	8.5
Fruit from allowance		
Dinner		
Broiled Sole with Brussels Sprouts (page 127)	190	9
2 bran muffins	136	4.5
Total	**1,016**	**42**

1,000-Calorie Menu for a Busy Housewife

Daily Allowance:

Fiber-Filler, 1 cup skim milk, 2 pieces of fruit	400	20

Midmorning

Late breakfast on half portion of Fiber-Filler and milk

Lunch

Three-Bean Salad with Egg (page 178)	200	8
Toasted whole-wheat English muffin	125	3.5

Afternoon Snack

Second portion of Fiber-Filler
Apple from allowance

Dinner

Bulgur Pilaf (page 195)	275	14

Evening Snack

Orange from allowance		
Total	**1,000**	**45.5**

1,000-Calorie Menu for a Vegetable Lover

	Calories	Grams of Fiber
Daily Allowance:		
Fiber-Filler, 1 cup skim milk, 2 pieces of fruit	400	20
Breakfast		
Half portion of Fiber-Filler with milk		
Orange from allowance		
Lunch		
Wintertime Special (page 126)	215	10
¼ cup low-fat yogurt	32	0
Diet soda	1	0
Late-Afternoon Snack		
Second portion of Fiber-Filler		
Fruit from allowance		
Dinner		
Baked Eggplant Casserole (page 150)	225	13
Small baked potato	120	5
Total	**993**	**48**

F-Plan for the Week

Here's the special seven-day F-Plan at the 1,250-calorie level. This is just a sample. There is an infinite range of variations that you'll develop as you go along.

MONDAY

This is a quick-and-easy selection for someone who doesn't like to bother too much.

	Calories	Grams of Fiber
Daily Allowance:		
Fiber-Filler, 1 cup skim milk, 2 pieces of fruit	400	20
Breakfast		
Cantaloupe (¼ of medium-sized melon)		
Half portion of Fiber-Filler with milk		
Lunch		
Chicken Salad Sandwich with Apple and Almonds (page 133)	235	7.5
Canned Apricots with Yogurt (page 209)	100	2.5

MONDAY

	Calories	Grams of Fiber

Afternoon Snack

Second portion of Fiber-Filler with
  milk
Orange from allowance
Tea or coffee

Dinner

	Calories	Grams of Fiber
Hamburger and Parsleyed Potato Dinner (page 143)	340	13.5
Strawberries with Almonds and Yogurt (page 208)	100	4
One glass red or white wine (4-ounce serving)	90	0
Total	**1,265**	**47.5**

TUESDAY

	Calories	Grams of Fiber
Daily Allowance:		
Fiber-Filler, 1 cup skim milk, 2 pieces of fruit	400	20
Breakfast		
Half portion of Fiber-Filler with milk from allowance		
Orange from allowance		
Lunch		
Roast Beef, Chickpea, and Feta Cheese Salad (page 178)	300	8.5
Fresh Peaches with Yogurt (page 210)	70	2.5
Coffee		
Dinner		
Broiled Chicken and Baked Potato Dinner (page 143)	315	11
Baked Apple Stuffed with Raisins and Nuts (page 213)	155	6

TUESDAY

	Calories	Grams of Fiber

TV Snack

Second portion of Fiber-Filler with
  milk
Apple from allowance

| | Total | 1,240 | 48 |

WEDNESDAY

	Calories	Grams of Fiber
Daily Allowance:		
Fiber-Filler, 1 cup skim milk, 2 pieces of fruit	400	20
Breakfast		
Half portion of Fiber-Filler with milk from allowance		
Orange from allowance		
Lunch		
Succotash Omelet (with 1 slice pumpernickel) (page 137)	325	9.5
2 tomato slices	20	1
Pear from allowance		
Afternoon Snack		
Second portion of Fiber-Filler with milk		
Tea		
Dinner		
Broiled Sole with Brussels Sprouts (page 127)	190	9

WEDNESDAY

	Calories	Grams of Fiber
Coleslaw with Apples and Raisins (page 177)	110	5.5
Banana	96	3
4-ounce glass white wine	90	0
Total	**1,231**	**48**

THURSDAY

	Calories	Grams of Fiber
Daily Allowance:		
Fiber-Filler, 1 cup skim milk, 2 pieces of fruit	400	20
Breakfast		
Half portion of Fiber-Filler with milk		
Orange from allowance		
Lunch		
Potato Soup (page 155)	80	4.5
Artichoke and Pimento Omelet (page 138)	300	11
Afternoon Snack		
Second portion of Fiber-Filler with milk		
Pear from allowance		
Coffee		
Dinner		
Bulgur Pilaf with Chicken (page 196)	435	14
½ cup low-fat cottage cheese	48	0
Total	**1,263**	**49.5**

FRIDAY

	Calories	Grams of Fiber
Daily Allowance:		
Fiber-Filler, 1 cup skim milk, 2 pieces of fruit	400	20
Breakfast		
Half portion of Fiber-Filler with milk		
2 plums from allowance		
Lunch		
Peanut Butter and Jam Sandwich (page 134)	290	8.5
Strawberry-Orange Compote (page 206)	60	2.5
Afternoon Snack		
Second portion of Fiber-Filler with milk		
Orange from allowance		
Dinner		
Whole-Wheat Spaghetti with Red Clam Sauce (page 201)	320	7.5

	Calories	Grams of Fiber
Tomato-Zucchini Salad (page 184)	60	3
Apricot-Grape Compote (page 209)	110	2.5
Total	**1,240**	**44**

SATURDAY

	Calories	Grams of Fiber
Daily Allowance:		
Fiber-Filler, 1 cup skim milk, 2 pieces of fruit	400	20
Breakfast		
Half portion of Fiber-Filler with milk		
Orange from allowance		
Lunch		
Hamburger and Vegetables (page 126)	310	9.5
Afternoon Snack		
Second portion of Fiber-Filler with milk		
Apple from allowance		
Tea		
Dinner		
Fresh Tomato Pizza with Mushrooms (page 190)	235	8.5

	Calories	Grams of Fiber
Mixed Vegetable and Cheese Salad (page 181)	125	5
4-ounce glass red wine	90	0
Blackberry Yogurt (page 214)	80	3
Total	**1,240**	**46**

SUNDAY

	Calories	Grams of Fiber
Daily Allowance:		
Fiber-Filler, 1 cup skim milk, 2 pieces of fruit	400	20
Breakfast		
Half portion of Fiber-Filler with milk		
Orange from allowance		
Lunch		
Chili con Carne (page 168)	205	7
Marinated Carrot Salad (page 184)	55	4
Raisin Bran Muffin (page 192)	85	3
Afternoon Snack		
Second portion of Fiber-Filler with milk		
Pear from allowance		
Coffee		
Dinner		
Okra and Pork Chop Dinner (page 148)	315	5

	Calories	Grams of Fiber
4-ounce glass red wine	90	0
Baked Apple (page 212)	95	4.5
Total	**1,245**	**43.5**

1,500-Calorie Menu

For the person who likes a glass of wine with dinner.

	Calories	Grams of Fiber
Daily Allowance:		
Fiber-Filler, 1 cup skim milk, 2 pieces of fruit	400	20
Breakfast		
Half portion of Fiber-Filler with milk		
Orange from allowance		
Lunch		
¼ cantaloupe (not from allowance)	40	1
Cornmeal Pancakes (page 194)	460	8
Afternoon Snack		
Second portion of Fiber-Filler with milk		
Banana from allowance		
Dinner		
Whole-Wheat Pasta with Chicken Livers (page 200)	415	8

	Calories	Grams of Fiber
Apricot-Grape Compote (page 209)	110	2.5
1 glass red or white wine (4-ounce serving)	90	0
Total	**1,515**	**39.5**

1,500-Calorie Menu

For the gourmet just starting on the diet.

	Calories	Grams of Fiber
Daily Allowance:		
Fiber-Filler, 1 cup skim milk, 2 pieces of fruit	400	20
Breakfast		
Half portion of Fiber-Filler with milk		
½ grapefruit from allowance		
Lunch		
Mexican Scrambled Eggs with Avocado and Kidney Beans (page 138)	375	9.5
Afternoon Snack		
Second portion of Fiber-Filler with milk		
Apple from allowance		
Tea		

	Calories	Grams of Fiber
Dinner		
Greek-Style Lamb Stew with Okra (page 150)	330	11
Canned Apricots with Yogurt (page 209)	100	2.5
TV Snack		
Graham Cracker Eggnog (page 203)	270	3
Total	**1,475**	**46**

The Metric System of Measurement

Spoonfuls	Milliliters
¼ teaspoon	1.25
½ teaspoon	2.5
¾ teaspoon	3.75
1 teaspoon	5
¼ tablespoon	3.75
½ tablespoon	7.5
¾ tablespoon	11.25
1 tablespoon	15

Ounces	
¼	7.5
½	15
¾	22.5
1	30

Cups	
¼	59
⅓	79
½	118
⅔	157
¾	177
1	236

Pints-Quarts-Gallons	
½ pint	237
1 pint	473
1 quart	946.3
1 gallon	3,785

Index

Bran, 9, 105
  Bran Flakes Plus, 120
  with breakfast cereal, 57
Bran Buds cereal, 64
Bran cereals, 58, 59, 105
Bran Chex cereal, 64
  with Sunflower Kernels, 120
Bran Flakes, 64, 120
Bran meal, 64
Bran muffins, 71
Brazil nuts, 64
Bread, 65
  for sandwiches, 130
Bread crumbs, 65
Breakfast, 55–58, 119–21
Breakfast cereals, 57–59, 119–21
  with bran, 57
Broccoli, 65
  Kasha with Beef (or Pork) and, 196–97
  Scallops with Squash and, 127
  Supreme, 126
Brown Lentil Soup, 159
Brown Rice Pilaf with Limas, 197
Brussels sprouts, 65
  Broiled Sole with, 127
Buckwheat groats (kasha), 65
Bulgur, 66
  Pilaf (Basic Recipe), 195
  Pilaf with Broiled Scrod, 196
  Pilaf with Chicken, 196
  Tabouleh (Lebanese Wheat Salad), 181
Burkitt, Denis, 103
Butter, 83
Buttermilk and Graham Crackers, 205

Cabbage, 66. *See also* Coleslaw
  and Fruit Salad, 175
Calcium, 45
Calories, 13–19, 39–42
  daily intake of, 39–42, 107
  dietary fiber and, 17–19
Cancer of the colon, 96–98
Cantaloupe, 66
Carrot(s), 66
  and Beet and Shrimp Salad, 180
  and Egg and Peanut Sandwich, 132
  -Peanut Butter, Homemade, 136

  and Peanut Butter and Raisin
    Sandwich, 134
  Salad, Marinated, 184–85
Casserole
  Chicken Noodle, 202
  Corn and Tomato, 148
  Eggplant, Baked, 150–51
  Kidney Bean and Pork, 168–69
Cauliflower, 66
Celery, 66
  Chicken Salad with Apple,
    Watercress, and, 175
Cellulose, 28
Cheese, 83–84
  Cottage, Baked Spinach and, 152
  and Cucumber Sandwich on Seven-
    Grain Bread, 132
  Escalloped Tomato with, 124
  Feta, and Roast Beef, and Chickpea
    Salad, 178–79
  Lentil Soup with, 160
  and Vegetable Salad, Mixes, 181
Cherries, 66–67, 118
Chestnuts, 67
Chewing, 9
  eating speed and, 22–23
  psychological satisfaction of, 26–27
Chicken, 80–81
  Broiled, and Baked Potato Dinner,
    143
  Broiled, and Limas, 127
  Bulgur Pilaf with, 196
  Coleslaw with Peas and, 178
  Corn and Bean Chowder with, 147
  Livers, Whole-Wheat Pasta with,
    200–201
  -Noodle Casserole, 202
  and Peanut Butter and Cranberry
    Relish Sandwich, 134
  Potato, Chicken, and Watercress
    Soup, 156
  in restaurants, 88
  Salad with Celery, Apple, and
    Watercress, 175
  Salad Sandwich with Apple and
    Almonds, 133
Chickpeas (garbanzos), 11, 67
  with Pork, 166
  and Roast Beef, and Feta Cheese
    Salad, 178–79